Professional Ethics and Law in the Health Sciences

Issues and Dilemmas

Professional Ethics and Law in the Health Sciences

ISSUES AND DILEMMAS

EDNA J. HUNTER
DANIEL B. HUNTER
EDITORS

ROBERT E. KRIEGER PUBLISHING COMPANY
Malabar, Florida
1984

Original Edition 1984
Based on previous edition Black, White and Gray

Printed and Published by
ROBERT E. KRIEGER PUBLISHING COMPANY, INC.
KRIEGER DRIVE
MALABAR, FLORDIA 32950

Printed in the United States of America

Library of Congress Cataloging in Publication Data

Black, white, and gray.
    Professional ethics and law in the health sciences.

    Reprint. Originally published: Black, white, and gray. 1st ed. San
Diego, Calif. : Hunter Publications, c1982.
    1. Mental health laws—United States—Addresses, essays, lectures.
2. Phychotherapists—Legal status, laws, etc.—United States— Addresses, essays, lectures. 3. Psychotherapy patients—United
States—Addresses, essays, lectures. 4. Psychotherapy ethics—Addresses, essays, lectures. I. Hunter, Edna J. II. Hunter, D.
(Daniel) III. Title.

KF3828.A75B54 1984	344.73'044	83-24819
ISBN 0-89874-711-2	347.30444	

PREFACE

Few textbooks on professional ethics and the law cover all the issues which may arise in a therapist's day-to-day practice; none cover them in depth. *Professional Ethics and Law in the Health Sciences* grew out of a graduate level course taught at United States International University in San Diego. The volume contains a potpourri of topics—legal, ethical, and philosophical—which can impact professionals in the field of health sciences, or at least cause them to stop and ponder from time to time. Not only do the chapters delve into the issues of human rights, they also touch upon the dilemmas of innovative psychotherapeutic techniques, dual relationships, conflictual loyalties, and divergent value systems. In the final chapter, a *Hippocratic Oath for Psychologists* is proposed. The views expressed are those of the authors, and not necessarily of the Editors. There is no guarantee as to the accuracy of laws cited nor interpretations given, since both laws and ethics are a function of time, place, and the individual's particular orientation.

Edna J. Hunter, Psychologist
Daniel B. Hunter, Attorney at Law

ACKNOWLEDGEMENTS

Our special note of thanks goes to *Dr. Joan F. Mayotte*, a private practitioner, for her assistance in chapter selection and preliminary editing of the volume; to *Nancy O'Neal* and *Patricia Tuning*, United States International University, for final editing, and to *Duncan Koler*, Calwestern University School of Law, for double-checking all legal cases cited. We must also thank our graduate students who struggled with a variety of legal and ethical dilemmas and made this volume possible.

CONTENTS

Family, Law, and Culture
An Overview of Parental Rights

CHAPTER 1

GAIL J. JOHNSON

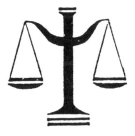

FAMILY, LAW, AND CULTURE AN OVERVIEW OF PARENTAL RIGHTS

1

Gail J. Johnson

The subject of this chapter is parental rights: their origin, character, evolution through time, place in culture, and the remarkable shift in their potency in colonial America. The opinions are those of the author.

Contemporary law will be examined in regard to parental rights with some views put forward about their future. As with all laws, there is a fairly straight line of development of parental laws from primitive laws, that is, the Babylonian and Hebrew Codes, to the Roman law. From Roman times onward, the ever-growing complexities of life and culture demanded more complex laws.

> Man has built up his law as he has built his whole civilization; by slow tentative and painful steps; testing the new, slow to reject the old. While this process, as we have seen, has not occurred at the same time in each department of the primitive law, it can also be observed in the law taken as a whole (Diamond, p. 141).

To introduce each code of the law, I will briefly describe their character, then the laws themselves, and finally, I will present my own analysis of perceived changes or additions in the law. As this will be original, there will be no sources cited. The material will be drawn from a long-time interest and study of world history and literature. Since primitive laws of parental rights are embedded in other kinds of law; i.e., inheritance, marriage, and property laws, I have tried to limit my scope to treating the subject firmly.

The first written laws that were concerned with the rights of parents over their offspring appeared in the Code of Hammurabi in 1914 B.C. Although King Hammurabi cited the sun god, Shamash, as his source of the law, he probably took liberally from Sumerian and Semitic laws of those city states' legislatures (Diamond, 1935). Parental rights did not exist in their own right and we must look to laws of property primarily to find regulations governing the relationships between father and offspring.

What is found is a stunning and awful power allowed a father over his children. A father was allowed to sell his children into slavery, either if the child displeased him in some way or in order to pay off debts (Diamond, 1935). A translation of the actual cuneiform states: "The debtor escapes from a personal liability by voluntarily delivering up some member of his family, either wife or child, to the creditor" (Driver & Miles, p. 209, Laws 117–119). "A debtor, the father, could also raise money by pledging or selling a dependent, but this pledge was not necessarily a life-long indenturing, only until the services of the child had raised the amount necessary or until the parent redeemed the child" (Driver & Miles, 1952).

Such action was not necessarily a popular practice. Most fathers were loath to sell their children, but the alternative was to sell himself into slavery and this was simply not a practical alternative. As head of the household, the father was the only member of the family who could conduct business and as he controlled all of the wealth of the family, he could not be spared. An analogous modern practice in Colonial America was the apprenticeship.

The Babylonian son could not hold property in his own name while he lived under his father's roof; his father had the rights to all of what a son might accrue (Diamond, 1935). If the son managed to obtain something of value, it became a part of his father's estate to be controlled by the father until the father died. At his death, the son might inherit what he had gained but, on the other hand, he might have to share it with other siblings and his mother.

The laws of inheritance were very complex indeed, involving legitimacy, slave children, divorced wives, and free women. Some of the bloodier codes of Hammurabi's law gave the father the right of life and death over his children and their mutilation, if he were so inclined (Diamond, 1935). "If a man strikes his father, his hand shall be cut off" (Driver & Miles, 1952, p.306). It is presumed that the father did the cutting in this matter for he judged all family matters, and the courts of this time did not interfere in family affairs. "If a son has denied his father, let the father shave him, put on him the mark of the slave and sell him" (Driver & Miles, 1952, p.306).

One might notice here that we are speaking of fathers and sons; mothers and daughters appear only in marriage laws as they apply to property. Like the son, any wealth a daughter might accrue went to the father's estate and, like the son, a daughter might be sold into slavery as a debt-slave. Where we find an additional proviso, however, is in the matter of the bride price. As any owner of goods expects a payment for them, fathers got good prices for their marriageable daughters. Usually, the daughter's consent was solicited but the father set her price according to how he valued her. If the daughter violated some part of the marriage contract, the bride price had to be returned to the husband; thus the father negotiated this matter very carefully (Diamond, 1935). Not citing his "witness," Diamond offered a Babylonian slice of life in the following:

> A father expects to get something for his daughter as she has to perform the duties of a wife and give birth to children. As these things are inflicted on the girl, the father must get something in compensation (Diamond, 1935, p.227).

Since the father had absolute authority, rights, and power over his children, he was also totally responsible for their conduct in the community. If they incurred a debt, he paid it. If they injured someone, he adjudicated the matter. He represented the family in all affairs and in all litigations (Diamond, 1935).

What strikes one about these laws is their severity and their sparseness. Only a very few laws are represented in the entire Code. Why might that be? As to their brevity and sparseness, I speculate that, as the family is the earlier social unit in man's historical evolution, custom and tradition were enough to govern relationships within the family.

Laws in the primitive world were legislated as the need for them arose and because the cultures of ancient Babylonia and Assyria were simple but growing, laws were simple and spare. As the culture became more complex, the laws become both more numerous and more complex. We shall see, throughout this history, that a culture is extremely well-measured by the quality, quantity and character of the law of that culture. An immensely interesting kind of relationship exists which deserves a far deeper study than space allows.

As to the absoluteness of the laws, I would speculate that it was in the best interests of the King and State to keep the family unit solid and unified. Harmony was the virture aimed at so that the affairs of the family would work as smoothly as the affairs of the state, both of which were managed with the absolute hand of the monarch.

Power was simply not delegated, for dissension would mean disunity and the breakdown of central authority. Severity followed from the nature of the times, as well. Physical survival was never assured and whatever promoted longer and better survival was deemed worthwhile.

The Hebrew Law: Pentateuch

During the Code of Hammurabi, which endured until about 400 B.C. and until the Roman Tablets of 485 B.C., another body of law was developing in a slow and organized manner. We find these laws in the Old Testament, a part of which was known as the Pentateuch. The entire Pentateuch includes the Book of Genesis up to and including Deuteronomy but that part of it which concerns us is only a few chapters in Exodus, 20–22. This is known as the Hebrew Code and is the oldest part of the Old Testament.

> Here the Hebrew, once a loose federation of tribes of mixed origin ... partly of Semitic, partly of Hittite, partly of Philistine and partly of other Indo European stock, have left us, embedded in the Bible, an invaluable Code of early law, probably influenced in its last days by contact with Babylonia (Diamond, 1935, p.15).

Between the Ten Commandments and the Hebrew Mosaic laws, we find some amazing secular laws. "Secular" must be qualified here. In my opinion, God is giving these laws to man and the religious sanctions for them are evident but the laws do not govern man's relationship to God, but to his fellow man.

After admonishing children to "Honor your father and your mother," in the Ten Commandments, a law I wish to return to a bit later, we find a new version of the old slave-debt laws.

> When a man sells his daughter as a slave, she shall not go out as male slaves do. If she does not please her master, who has designated her for himself, then he shall let her be

redeemed; he shall have no right to sell her to a foreign people (Exodus 21:7).

Let me offer an analysis of this interesting law. We see its obvious similarity to Hammurabi's law of slave-debt and the right of a father to sell his child, but here daughters are treated differently from sons. The daughter "goes out" of slavery in a different manner. She may be redeemed as a son might be but she cannot be sold to a foreign people. That is a very interesting addition. Why was it added? I speculate that, as God gave the Land of Plenty to his Chosen People, it was His intention that they remain there and populate it. He admonishes them to "be fruitful and multiply." If a daughter were sold into a foreign land, she could not be redeemed easily but, more importantly, she would not bear Hebrew children in the Chosen Land. The population would suffer that loss.

Another consideration is the same as I observed in regard to Hammurabi's Code: that the family must retain its unity and cohesiveness and if a daughter were sold away, this structure would be weakened. The family had to be maintained as a strong, fighting unit to preserve its gains and to increase the tribe.

Going back for a moment to the Commandment cited earlier, let me complete the quotation, for now it gains new significance.

Honor your father and your mother, that your days may be long in the land which the Lord, your God, gives you (Exodus 20:12).

Extrapolating from this, we see, when joined with the other law discussed, that *if* they failed to honor their father and their mother, they might indeed be sold into slavery and *not* enjoy their days in the land which their God had given them. As this law is immediately followed by that applying to the daughter's situation, I surmise that sons, unlike daughters, might be sold to a foreign peoples.

The next law which touches upon parent-child relations is:

Whoever strikes his father or his mother shall be put to death (Exodus 21:15).

Followed by:

Whoever curses his father or his mother shall be put to death (Exodus 21:15).

These three laws are all related to governing family relationships in the Hebrew Code. What I have noted about them is, first, that mothers and daughters now are a profound part of a law which hitherto was entirely male.

Recall that the Hammurabi Code mentioned only that a man could sell his son into slavery; the daughter was not mentioned. Now, also, a mother may not be offended by her children, by *law*. Mothers, in Hammurabi's Code were only mentioned in regard to inheritance laws. Now they command honor, respect, and are protected from the criminal acts of their children.

This brings us to the subject pronoun, "whoever." Comparing this with "If a man strikes his father . . ." we see that Hebrew law does not specify male or female; it does not discriminate. Presumably a daughter who strikes her mother might be killed as well as a son. It seems remarkable to me that women have made themselves an essential part of the law at so early a date.

Another distinction that occurs to me here is the difference in proportion between crime and punishment. The distance has grown and what makes it the more remarkable is that the law of Talio was very much in effect during these times and is recorded later in the Pentateuch. After pronouncing punishment for jostling a pregnant women who miscarries, the command continues:

> . . . if any harm follows then you shall give life for life, eye for eye, tooth for tooth, hand for hand, foot for foot, burn for burn, wound for wound, stripe for stripe . . (Exodus 21:23).

Talio, the great equalizer before the law, does not apply for crimes against a parent and this suggests, more than ever, the respect and honor due to parents and their immense prestige in ancient Hebrew civilization. Certainly the whole character of Hebrew law is more severe than Hammurabi's and more primitive as well.

This presents us with another interesting consideration. The spirit of both laws seems different. In Hammurabi, the sense is that a man may exert his discretion over the law: he may do as he pleases and it is his prerogative not to sell his son or cut off his hand. But the law of the Hebrews does not suggest this leeway. A man is *obliged* to punish an offender. And we know from reading the rest of the Old Testament, that fathers did indeed kill their offspring for offenses. It seems to me that parents by that time now had a duty to observe the law and this duty was not just to their society, but to God, and an "awful" God at that.

In general, one could say that these laws were more primitive than those of Hammurabi, for life among the Hebrew tribes was just barely settled from nomadic to agrarian. The laws were fewer and they were far more simple even than the Hammurabi Code. In fact, Babylonia had become a commercial world power while the Hebrews were still wandering around in the wilderness. Although it is not shown in the laws of parental rights to any great extent, the laws governing commerce and contracts were highly sophisticated and complex.

Except for the recognition of women in the Hebrew law, that law took a long step backward with the Pentateuch. These laws lack humanism. The God of the Old Testament certainly has not been described as a humane figure historically, but theology is not the proper subject of this present chapter.

Roman Law

The origins of Roman Law are mysterious and much contended. Some scholars have felt that religious and mythological sources presented law to the Roman peoples and that priests mediated its promulgation. Others have felt that law came to Rome by way of its colonies in Greece who had gotten it from the Hittites who had gotten it from Babylon. Still others cite the Cretan Codes of Gortyn as a source in 450 B.C. As Rome had colonies all over the known world, the origins may have been multiple.

One problem is that the Greeks and Egyptians, both brilliant civiiizations in law, recorded these laws on papyrus and as that material is perishable, their laws were lost. But word of mouth may have carried law to the great Capital of Rome. What we do see is a profound similarity between Roman and Babylonian law; thus there is internal evidence. The famous Twelve Tablets appeared in the First Century B.C. and developed into a tool which constituted one of Rome's greatest achievements as well as that of Western man (Encyclopedia Britannica, Volume 6).

In our area of exploration, the doctrine of paterfamilias commands our attention first and foremost. In a modified fashion, it will dominate family law for centuries to come and indeed is a distinguishing characteristic of English common law and American colonial law.

> The family is the legal unit of society. Its head, the pater-familias, is the only full person known to the law. His children of whatever age, though they are citizens and therefore have rights in public law, are subject to his un-fettered power of life and death (Nicholas, 1962, p.65).

We have noted earlier that fathers had the power of life and death over their offspring and while this is demonstrated in Roman law, we begin to see that the State will restrict this right. This is perhaps one of the first intrusions of the State into the domain of family relationships. At the end of the second century, the law stated that a father could kill his son only if he first consulted with a council of advisors or tribunal and that the son must exhibit profoundly bad conduct to warrant such a punishment.

The father might then proceed, but only with the consent of the tribunal. An oft-quoted case, recorded in English common law and also in American colonial law, cites Hadrian punishing a father by banishing him because the father had murdered the son for committing incest with his step-mother (Nicholas, 1962, 67). What we observe is that the law was becoming more "civilized" and more humane as time progressed and as culture absorbed the qualities of Christianity.

> Social habits were changing and the over-indulgent parent was replacing the stern father of an earlier day, so that, by the end of the classical period, the power of life and death was probably obsolete—except for the practice, common in the ancient world, of exposing newborn babies; this was made criminal in 374 A.D. (Nicholas, 1962, p.80).

As a father might, with consent, kill his son and his slave (the two are almost alike under the paterfamilias doctrine), he could also sell them. Both son and slave were considered property to be disposed of as the paterfamilias wished. As we saw in primitive law, the father always reserved the right to redeem a son he had sold and now even his rights to sell that son and to redeem him again were restricted by the law, another encroachment that signals what is in the offing.

A father, according to the Twelve Tablets, could only sell his son three times and then that son was to be free forever (Nicholas, 1962). Oddly enough, a daughter and a grandchild could only be sold once. Justinian finally swept the whole practice of reselling and redeeming away and left only the essential: that a magistrate enter the proceeding on a court record.

A good deal of attention was given to laws of inheritance under Roman law. As Rome expanded and became a great commercial power, wealth came into the hands of citizens, merchants, and politicians. Indeed even the lowly soldier of the Republic could be granted large land plots in return for his service. The laws governing what a son might expect from his father in terms of property by inheritance came under the heading of *patria potestas* (in the power of the father). Like Babylonian law, only the father could own property and whatever a son acquired belonged to his father alone (Nicholas, 1962). However, a softening of the law is observed in practice in that the father most often allowed his son the use of what that son had acquired but the father could remove it whenever the mood fell upon him.

Interestingly, a father could not disinherit his son except by permission of a council or tribunal (Nicholas, 1962). A son might chose not to inherit (in the case of debts, for example). This was to insure the continuity of succession. Indeed, if a Roman will failed to name an heir, succession was considered invalid (Nicholas, 1962). Again, to an exceptional degree, the State was allowed by law to interfere in the matters of the family, especially where money or property was concerned.

The inheritance laws are so complex that it is difficult to follow them into the maze of legal tangles. Divorced women and their children had different privileges; slave women and their children had provisions; adopted sons were treated differently, as were bastard sons.

Besides noting the interference of the State into the family, several other aspects of Roman law must be studied. First, we see that there is public law and private law for the first time, but we also note that public law superseded private law in at least two matters: life and death of children and inheritance.

What was missing in the law as it was stated were punishments attached to various crimes. Heretofore, in statements of law, both the crime and its punishment came together within the statement. This suggests that a third voice determined punishment, the courts or tribunals. This was not the case in primitive law.

Another difference in Roman law was that it was almost exclusively concerned with property and the distribution of property by selling or inheritance, where children were concerened. The law lacked the blood and guts of primitive law; matters of honor were not the concern of the law. The law had become more abstract; less was left to a father's whim and more to a benevolent court.

But once again, there were not, proportionately, many laws governing family relationships. The authority of the father was absolute and as he decided and controlled what went on in his household, there was less need for codified law. The man was the law.

Anglo-Saxon Law

As there is very little left to us of secular, Anglo-Saxon law, our remarks here will be brief. The period is only important as a link between Roman and Common Law.

First, we must jump forward in time from the fall of Rome, in 200 A.D. to about 600 A.D. As the Empire began to crumble, its laws became both chaotic and stale. Nothing of excellence was added; however, some Germanic fragments were tacked on.

In England, where Roman colonies were billeted until 436 A.D., Roman law governed Romans, but local, tribal law governed the "barbarians," that is, the Angles, Saxons, Goths, Picts, Burgundians, Scots, and Jutes. If laws were required to adjudicate an affair between a Roman and a barbarian, Roman law took precedence.

> The Roman colonies continued to live under the Roman law of the province; the barbarians ruled their subjects of their own race under native rules. Yet the prestige of Rome was still such that the barbarian kings were often content to own her over-lordship. These peoples had adopted much of Roman civilization as well as Christianity and when they produced written law, it was law much influenced by contact with Rome (Diamond, 1935, p.16).

Although the time of the Anglo-Saxon law was closer chronologically to modern times, the character of the law was a giant step backward. Tribal law, of course, cannot rival the laws of the great empires but another important fact must come into play here, that reading and writing were skills nonexistent for the law peoples of England. The Church controlled literature and law which was written in Latin. Since Canon law is very complex and regulates affairs within the Church, I have chosen not to include it. The condition just described maintained until the 11th Century. Unfortunately, we are left with little more than scraps.

What we do have is a fragment from the Code of Euric which was written down between 466–485 A.D. when he ruled the West Goths. Nothing more is discovered until the more famous Dooms (laws) of Aethelbert, 600 A.D. They are our primary source for this period.

> The spirit of the law was that physical control meant legal jurisdiction and, conversely, jurisdiction meant power (Diamond, 1935, p.332).

Does this translate into laws of parental rights? I think it does if we consider that when matters of jurisdiction come into play, one begins to consider hierarchies: *who* has control of what, or *who* has control of *how much*. Indeed hierarchies were the natural framework for this feudal period simply because we have a king with a court and clerics and knights and squires and commoners.

Once again we see that the law reflects culture, for Anglo-Saxon law was arranged according to the social hierarchy. The laws were set down according to the social class of the person against whom a crime was committed. Clerics came first after the person of the King (Diamond, 1935, p.65).

The dominant theme of the law as stated in the Dooms was that each man, like the King, was compensated when his own peace was breached (Diamond, 1935). No more specific laws are given that would touch upon our subject.

A corollary, however, reminds us of the paterfamilias doctrine and Hammurabi, in that the father is solely responsible to the chieftain of his tribe for members of his family. When conflict breaks out between two families, that chieftain will judge the matter; when a conflict breaks out among family members, the father will judge the matter. When conflict breaks out among tribes within his kingdom, a king will judge the matter, and so up the hierarchy we go.

Law was not really a primary concern for the tribes of England during this period. Men were too busy keeping their heads to use them in manufacturing codes of conduct. Boundaries shifted constantly as warfare ensued. Peacetime was the exception. It is no wonder then that "jurisdiction" characterizes what little we have of law at this time. As I stated elsewhere, laws are created as they are needed by a culture and each tends to reflect the other. Times were chaotic, as was the law, and this situation continued to exist until Henry II managed to bring England under one central authority in the 11th Century. Until then, law waited in the wings while war was centre-stage.

English Common Law

With Henry II and peace, Englishmen could now pause, collect themselves, and turn their attention to matters of language, literature, and law. A revival of classical literature unearthed the laws of Justinian, which had lain around in monastery libraries for centuries, waiting for their time. Now that lawmen had the tools and the need for further laws (they could read and write by this time), this was the time. Increased population, expansion into the world outside England, commerce and the rise of the middle or merchant class, required that there be some laws to govern these areas. In fact, with regard to law the British Empire of the 11th through the 13th Centuries was not unlike that of Justinian's reign in 200 B.C. The legal capabilities of each culture were equal (Diamond, 1935).

In the English Common law of the 13th Century, for the first time we find that parental rights are treated as a part of the law in and for themselves; they were not a part of property or inheritance or marriage laws. In his *Commentaries*, Blackstone (1765), arranged the laws governing the domestic scene into three categories: laws governing duties of children toward their parents, laws governing duties of parents toward their children, and the powers of parents over their children. All of these laws fall under the overall category of "Laws Dealing with Persons." Simply from this fact, we see how far the law had come in its specificity from old tribal law. But the organization still reflects something of that ancient period.

Another important feature to note in the law is that parents now had *duties*. Nowhere in law previously had duties been set down; they had always been the obligations of children, not parents. While we saw in Roman law that the State was willing to encroach upon the rights of parents in certain matters, this trend was expanded in English Common Law. Parental power was more limited and ascribing duties to parents was the first step in this process. But what were these duties?

The duties of 13th Century parents were "to maintain, educate and to protect" their offspring (Blackstone, 1765, p.447). Custom had provided for these offices previously and we might well ask ourselves why they were now matters of law? I would venture that because of the changing times in Britain, the nature of family life was changing as well. As the feudal system was breaking down, absolute rule was also crumbling around the edges. On the political scene, despotism, so enjoyed previously by English kings, gave way to legislation by King and Parliament. In the family, the father was restrained as well, in that duty restricted his rights. This condition did not develop because *children* now had rights. Indeed they would have to wait centuries more for this miracle; it simply meant that the State would control family matters in a way they had never done before.

As the absolute powers of King and father declined, we see that more law was required and more specific law, at that. Elsewhere I stated that when power is absolute, law is simple and brief. The opposite also obtains; when power is not absolute, law is complex and abundant. In Common Law there was a tremendous increase in the number and in the complexity of laws governing family affairs.

One factor did not change in the law, but it was modified: children continued to be regarded as property. Note what Blackstone wrote: ". . . every man has, or ought to have, by the laws of society, a power over his own property: and . . . natural right obliges him to give a necessary maintenance to children; but what is more than that, they have no other right to, than as it is given them by the favour of their parents, or the positive constitutions of the municipal law (Blackstone, 1765, p.448)."

Here Blackstone, commenting on the law, set the cornerstone upon which domestic law was built for centuries to come. With rights came duties. The father had the right to his children for they were his property, but he had the duty to maintain them because they were his property. As a corollary, we see that a father was *not* obliged to maintain lazy children and he had the right to disinherit his children. What we have, in essence, was giving rights with one hand of the law and giving out duties or restrictions of those rights with the other. The law was saying, "See here, you must do this but we will make it easier for you for you don't have to do this other."

> For the policy of our laws, which are ever watchful to promote industry, did not mean to compel a father to maintain his idle and lazy children in ease and indolence; but thought it unjust to oblige a parent, against his will, to provide them with superfluities and other indulgences of fortune" (Blackstone, 1765, p.448).

The spirit of the law is almost paternalistic, almost apologetic. It is, indeed, a far cry from the harsh laws of the Hebrew or the bland but reasonable voice of the Roman law.

The next duty of the father, to educate his child, follows this same spirit. While the father must see to it that his child learn to read and write, he need not, if the child elects to be a Roman Catholic. Then the child is on his own. The father has the right to determine what kind of education his child will have.

Protection is the third obligation of the father. In primitive law, we saw that the father was responsible to society for crimes and debts of his children. In common law, this held true as well, but the obligation was qualified somewhat.

> A parent may, by our law, maintain and uphold his children in their law suits without being guilty of the legal crimes of maintaining quarrels. A parent may also justify an assault and battery in defense of his children. (Blackstone, 1965, p.450).

The parent is not culpable as he was in earlier law nor is he liable for debt. What is interesting is that physically, he can defend his children, hurting another, and not be considered guilty of assault and battery.

Without hesitating further, let us go on to a consideration of parental rights or "powers" as Blackstone calls them. If we are to impose obligations on a parent, we must give him some rights which are related to these obligations. These powers are meant to help the parent carry out his duties more effectively and they also serve as recompense for his "care and trouble in the faithful discharge of it" (Blackstone, 1765, p.453).

The first right a parent possesses is that of discipline.

> The power of a parent by our English laws is much more moderate (than the Roman); but still sufficient to keep the child in order and obedience. He may lawfully correct his child, being under age, in a reasonable manner; for this is for the benefit of his education" (Blackstone, 1765, p.452).

The English Common Law had great faith in the workings of parental affection and the thought that a parent might unnaturally brutalize his child was unthinkable. Natural law was a very strong force during this era and upon it was built social law. Both governed the delicate workings of family relationships. But, as we will see, the law was naive in this respect.

In matters of property rights, English Common law was more lenient than the Roman law, upon which it is based. The father could realize benefits and profits, such as rents, from property owned by his child (minor), but when that child reached his majority, the father had to give him an account of how these monies had been used. The father had the benefit of his child's own labor while he lived with him but, "this is no more than he is entitled to from his apprentices or servants" (Blackstone, 1765, p.453). The spirit of the paterfamilias remained but the absolute powers did not. What the child owned was the child's but his father watched over it while the child was a minor. What the child *earned* was another matter completely.

The subject of apprenticeship is seen here for the first time and demands a remark or two. We see that a father cannot sell his son into slavery as the primitive and Roman fathers were allowed to do, but he could arrange an apprenticeship for that son, a term of training for which the father was recompensed. The son had little to say about the matter, but had to serve out his time and give up his earnings nonetheless.

Another right of the father had to do with marriage. A son or daughter could not marry without the consent of the father. To the English way of thinking, this requirement protected the child from entering into an alliance with "the snares of artful and designing persons." This was also meant to facilitate settling a son or daughter properly in life by preventing the ill consequences of too early a marriage. After the child reached majority, this right, as all rights of the parent, was no longer in effect.

Other rights of the parent were construed to maintain a modicum of power over the child even after death. The design of the father's will was one of these means as well as the appointment of a guardian for the child or a tutor who held power *in loco parentis*.

This superb body of law was firmly based upon the best of Justinian's humane law. The law in fifteen centuries had become a more flexible tool for governing human affairs. It became more benevolent, more paternalistic, but also more naive.

It carried with it a sensivity not found in earlier law anywhere, and for this we can look to the driving force of Christian Humanism more than to any other consideration. The important, over-riding feature of this law was that the State or Crown, if you will, now interferes in family relationships and encroaches upon the absolute rights of the father. Unhappily, women seem to have sunk back into obscurity once again and remained there for many years.

For the sake of perspective, let us see what was *not* in the law. A father no longer had the power of life and death over his child. This was totally new. A father no longer dealt with his son's property with impunity. A father now had rights *and* duties. It was really quite remarkable how far the law had come.

American Colonial Law

As the English colonists began to settle themselves into their respective places along the Atlantic seaboard in the 16th Century, the question of law became a moot one. Once their allegiance to England was breached, they abjured all things English except tea, and they also refused to use English Common law. Most colonists had suffered enormously from it, especially in matters of religious preference. We should remember that persons convicted of crimes were routinely shipped over to the colonies to work out their period of indenturement. Thus, "they did not claim or desire the common law" (Encyclopedia Britannica, Vol. 6, p.757).

The colonists were forced back upon their own resources, and each colony created its own bodies of law according to its own needs and desires. But since most colonists were not versed in law and had little education beyond reading and writing, chaos followed. With few lawyers, fewer judges and no schools of law, the embroilment was so severe that finally the colonists saw the futility of their efforts.

> In the 18th Century, common law was adopted and colonial statutes disallowed as law became more central and more professional (Encyclopedia Britannica, Vo. 6, p.758).

As we see from my primary source for this period, James Kent (1884), Colonial law followed fairly directly from the English Common law and the trend of interference by the State (or Crown) pervaded more and more insistently. The State gave itself this power to work in its own behalf for the sake of the common good.

As parental rights were more and more restricted, we might hope that children's rights would be increasing, but that, sadly enough, had to wait for a few hundred years. The State was taking up the slack left by the encroachment, but children were somewhat better off than they had been previously.

What we observe in Kent (1884) is that the duties of the parent outweighed his rights and that a great shift had occurred as the Common law traversed the Atlantic. As before, duty and right were inextricably woven into the same cloth. For the sake of convenience, I will list them with brief notes following:

(1) It was the duty of the parent to maintain a child until that child provided for itself. Normally, but not always, that age cut-off was twenty-one. Rather poetically the law read:

> Under the thousand pains and perils of human life, the home of the parents is to the children a sure refuge from evil, and a consolation in distress. In the intenseness, the lively touches, and unsubdued nature of parental affection, we discern the wisdom and goodness of the great Author of our being, and Father of Mercies (Kent, 1884, p.237).

The religious coloration here reminds us that it was the Puritans and other religious zealots who fled England to settle in the new world. The authority of the law was not natural law, as we saw in Common law, but Divine Law. The flavor of the Hebrew tradition was faint, but nevertheless there.

(2) If a parent were not capable of maintaining his child, the township would do so, but if he chose not to, he could be sued for maintainance for necessities and for schooling. While Common law inferred that a father would be punished for failing to maintain his child, here we see clear proof that a third party, the court, would make certain that a child was cared for by his parent. Even if the child's estate happened to be greater than his parent's, the father was still liable, if he had the ability to support the child.

But Kent (1884) adds, if that were the case, the law relaxed somewhat. The court decided these matters by the circumstances which attached to the case. Of course, what the court wanted to avoid was pauper children running about loose in the streets, children who would become a burden on the township or the State. In this respect, it was not necessarily for the welfare of the child that the State was so concerned; it was for its own purse.

(3) The father was not bound by the contracts or debts of his son, even for necessities (Kent, 1884).

This law compares clearly with Common law. What constitutes "necessities" was left up to a third party, the court, to determine. We see, more and more, that this third party intervened in determining domestic matters and in limiting the parental privilege.

(4) If a father forced a child from home by "severe usage," he was liable for his necessities. (This was the first recognition that a father might, indeed, use his child badly and the naivete of the common law was somewhat lifted).

(5) A father was entitled to the custody of his children and to the value of their labors and services as the consequence of his obligation for their maintenance and, in some qualified degree, for their education (Kent, 1884).

Nothing much has changed in this law except that the qualification for education was not strictly stated.

(6) A father could obtain the custody of his child by writ of habeas corpus when the child was improperly detained from him but the child's inclination was solicited and if he were mature enough in judgment, he controlled the father's right to custody. The court had the final judgment (Kent, 1884).

This view was strikingly modern. For the first time, the powers of a child were greater than those of his father over him. The child could decide whether or not he wished to continue living under his father's roof or if he wished the court to find another roof for him.

In matters of education, the law read:

(1) The education of children in a manner suitable to their station and calling is another branch of parental duty, of imperfect obligation generally in the eyes of the municipal law, but of very great importance to the welfare of the state (Kent, 1884, p.244)

There were several loopholes in this law that a father could take advantage of. For one thing, education was not defined as reading or writing skills. It might well have been an apprenticeship in which a child learned a trade. That probably would have satisfied the state, for the "station" of such a child was probably a poor one and it was better that he be able to earn his living than to read and write. If a child could not support himself, the state was obliged to take care of him and that was *not* in its best interest.

Continuing:

> Without some preparation made in youth for the sequel of life, children of all conditions would probably become idle and vicious when they grow up, either from the want of good instruction and habits . . . or from want of rational and useful occupation (Kent, 1884, p.245)

We have all heard of the Puritan ethic from which America sprang. Here it is in full force. If a child wasn't occupied, he would surely go to perdition.

What is interesting about this insistence upon education, no matter what its calibre, is that education became compulsory. It did not matter whether the parents undertook to teach the child themselves, as many did. What was required was that the child know how to read and write or how to maintain himself when he came of age. In community law, we find that each township of 50 families or more was obliged to offer its children a school in which they might obtain an education. Furthermore, if parents refused to teach their children or allow them to go to the school, the selectmen of the community were obliged to remove the children from their parents and place them with masters who would see to their education. This was the case, for instance, in Massachusetts in 1647 (Kent, 1884, p.250).

Besides preventing paupers from flooding the dole system, Kent pointed out education is necessary to create the scholarly men much needed to govern the nation.

> . . . it is the higher schools that must educate those accomplished men who are fit to lead the public councils and to be entrusted with the guardianship of our laws and liberties and who can elevate the character of the nation (Kent, 1884, p.263).

In case something was left out of law which had to do with parental obligation, a blanket law was devised to fill in the gaps.

> The remaining branch of parental duty consists in making competent provisions, according to the circumstances of the father, for the welfare and settlement of the child; but this duty is not susceptible of municipal regulation and left to the dictates of reason and natural affection (Kent, 1884, p.203).

We should pause for a moment to see what had been omitted in these parental duties. One was protection. Unlike the common law, which was quite detailed in this, a child was no longer protected by his father. More than likely, the state had assumed that burden. Another law was omitted; a father need not leave his child anything in his will. He could leave everything to a stranger, if he wished to do so.

Although the number of duties that a parent was obliged to observe were actually less than in Common law, there were more specific regulations than previously, especially in the matter of the duty to educate a child. Education, in this New World, had taken on great significance and import.

But, like the Common law, the state saw that if it were to require parents to fulfill certain duties, it must offer some kind of compensation. Parents were thus rewarded by having authority over their children:

> ... and in support of that authority, a right to exercise of such discipline as may be requisite for the discharge of their sacred trust. This is the true foundation of parental power (Kent, 1884, p.264).

Unlike other powers we shall examine shortly, the state did not qualify this right. It only called for "moderate correction under the exercise of a sound discretion." Like Common law, the state assumed that parents had sound discretion.

(2) The parent had the right of custody of his child but if that parent were found wanting, the custody reverted elsewhere by the determination of the court. (Kent did not go into detail regarding this law and that is a shame for such material would be interesting indeed.)

(3) The parent had the right to earnings of his apprenticed child and that child's services.

An interesting note here is that if a daughter were seduced by her master while apprenticed to him, it was felt that the father could sue that master for depriving the father of his daughter's services. This followed, whether the girl was made pregnant or not! However, if seduction were a part of the contract, then the father could not sue. While this "law" offends anyone's gentility and was an outrage, it was common practice for fathers to sell their daughters into prostitution if they had to—better that than be a pauper! Anything, including her virtue and well-being could be the price the state was willing for the family to pay to keep that child off the dole.

(4) The final right of the parent to have custody of the estate of his minor child remained.

The father could take the rents and profits of his child until that child was 21 or emancipated. Unlike Common law, in Colonial law the father was not obliged to give an accounting of how he had used this estate to the child when he or she reached 21. Presumably, he could do as he wished with it.

In summary, then, there were only four rights which remained more or less intact at the end of the Colonial period and at the beginning of the modern era: the parents still had the right to educate his child as he saw fit; he had custody of his children; he had the right to profits from the child's estate; and, finally, he had the right to discipline his child as he saw fit.

Modern Law

Because Modern Law is still in a state of tremendous flux, the final word about it is forthcoming. The material I have used in this formulation comes mainly from Clark, whose book, *The Law of Domestic Relationships* (1968), although the most comprehensive, was not the most recent available, especially in the area of the parental right to discipline children. My remarks must necessarily fall a little short of an up-to-the-minute accounting.

Let us begin by examining the four rights remaining to parents at the close of the Colonial period and how these rights have altered. The first, the right of the parent to educate his child as he saw fit, was changed radically by the advent of compulsory education.

The limits imposed on the parent earlier stipulated only that the parent was obliged to make certain his child could read and write so that that child could gain employment as an adult and not become a ward and burden to the state. The laws of compulsory education have laid a further restriction upon parents. School-age children are required by law to attend school whether their parents teach them to read and write at home or not.

> All children within certain age limits are subject to state statutes compelling their education. Compulsory education laws have uniformly been sustained against various charges that individual liberties guaranteed by the Constitution have been violated (Houlgate, 1980, p.23).

From this quotation, we see that attendance at school has replaced the requirements of reading and writing.

Compulsory education came out of the Industrial Revolution and is an interesting phenomenon because it was not the best interests of the child that determined the quality of the law; it was the common good that prevailed. Almost by accident the child was rescued from the workbench and sent off to school. This ruling occurred because the work market became glutted with young children, and employment for adults became jeopardized.

In order to maintain full employment for mature males and females, something had to be done with children. Thus the State, in its benevolence, sent them off to school (Lecture, Keasey, D.B., University of California, Riverside, Summer 1979). Since these children, it was assumed, would be capable of supporting themselves after the eighth grade, the State would not have their care in their hands.

Note that the parents' rights had narrowed as had their choices for their child's education. Only rarely, in cases when religious training would be deeply interrupted, did the law allow the parent more than a choice between public and private education.

The second right of the parent, his right to the wages and services of his child, has undergone even more dramatic changes over the years. This movement began in the 1800s when the difference between a child and an adult was first recognized by law in England. In 1802 the first Child Labor law was enacted which prevented a child from working in the cotton mills for over twelve hours a day. Unfortunately, this law was not enforced. The Factory Act of 1833 prohibited a child under the age of nine from working, and restricted children under 14 to 48 hours of work per week. The Benthamite Doctrine of 1834 regulated conditions in the poor houses which were intentionally kept unbearable so that few persons would go on relief.

Oliver Twist was written, in fact, to call attention to this deplorable situation. In 1842, the Royal Commission issued a report that children as young as five were working 16 hours a day in coal mines. The House of Lords prohibited boys and girls under 10 from working in the mines for any length of time.

It is clear that children needed interference from the State in the matter of child labor. Many of them died from overwork and exploitation by their parents. In America the statement regulating child labor expressed this sentiment:

> Child labor laws . . . are founded upon the principle that the supreme right of the State to the guardianship of children controls the natural rights of the parent when the welfare of society or of the children themselves conflicts with parental rights (Abbott, 1938, p.325).

The encroachment was complete; the State had found it necessary to protect a minor from his parents. A great hue and cry went up against this legislation. Parents felt their rights were violated and their poverty assured. "A Communist Plot" was blamed by some for the passage of this legislation, but the court held that:

> It is not an undue restriction of the rights of the parent to the labor of the child, assuming that he has such a right, when opposed to the general welfare. It does not close to him all fields of employment for his child, but only those in factories and manufacturing establishments . . . (Abbott, 1938, p.325).

California statute prohibiting employment of children under the age of 14 included "any mercantile institution, office, laundry, manufactory, workshop, restaurant, or apartment house."

The third right, the right to discipline his child as he saw fit, has become a hotbed of controversy in recent years as children began turning up in X-ray units with mysterious fractures. The profundity and wide-spread nature of this horror set the United Nations into action, and in 1960 the General Assembly issued a document that has been enormously important in the field of domestic law. *The United Nations Declaration of the Rights of the Child* came into being. The ninth principle applies directly to child abuse.

> The child shall be protected against all forms of neglect, cruelty and exploitation. He shall not be the subject of traffic, in any form (U.N. General Assembly Resolution 1386 (XIV), November 20, 1959, supplemented 1960).

For the first time a child's rights limit those of his parent insofar as he is protected by the State from inhumane treatment by that parent. The United Nations further stipulated that the child is entitled to:

> ... special protection ... to enable him to develop physically, mentally, morally, spiritually and socially in a healthy and normal manner and in conditions of freedom and dignity (U.N. General Assembly, Principle Two, November 20, 1959, supplemented 1960).

Child abuse and child neglect are recognized as very complex issues and all ramifications of the problem cannot be described here. In fact, laws are still pending on this issue and the final word has certainly not been spoken. What we do have are laws regulating the reporting of child abuse or neglect that are pervasive. All professionals who encounter or suspect a case of child abuse must report it to Protective Services authorities. This includes doctors, mental health professionals, nurses, teachers, and lawyers, in some states, although states vary on these requirements (Schwitzgebel & Schwitzgebel, 1980).

In the Federal Child Abuse Prevention and Treatment Act of 1974 child abuse refers to "physical or mental injury, sexual abuse, negligent treatment or maltreatment of a child" (Schwitzgebel & Schwitzgebel, 1980, p.166). By definition, child abuse is "the intentional use of force resulting in physical injury serious enough to endanger the health or life of the child" .... and is a criminal offense in all states. Neglect is defined as "inadequate child care of a physical nature, and sometimes to the failure to insure conditions for positive, social-psychlogical development" (Schwitzgebel & Schwitzgebel, 1980, p.165).

Part of the problem in child abuse legislation is that law is most often based on previous law and decisions, and for this reason absolute parental rights which have endured for two thousand and more years of recorded history simply will not give way easily or quickly. It was, in fact, on the shirt-tails of a law preventing cruelty to animals that any legislation for children was ever devised. In 1824, the National Society for the Prevention of

Cruelty to Animals and Children finally acted in behalf of these subjects. In New York, in 1874, the famous case of Mary Ellen, an abused child, finally shook the attention of the public. But we can see how long it had been in coming and how long it may be until really good and inclusive laws prevail.

My final consideration is the right of the parent to the custody of his child. Of this area, Foster says:

> The last century also saw the demise of the common law notion that the father always should have custody of his children (if he wanted them) and the emergence of the vague "best interests of the child" standard (Foster, 1974, p.5).

Clark was more specific:

> ... the courts have been far too often influenced by the notion that the parent has a "right" to his child. This idea carries echoes of the law of property. The child is treated as chattel. A proper decision on parental rights should take into account not merely the natural parents "rights" but the extent to which he has failed to perform his parental obligations (Clark, 1968, pp. 630–631).

And so, the final privilege of a parent, to have a child in his custody and to care for him, was challenged in Modern Law. How the ancients would have been amazed by this infringement! But the "times, they are a-changing." In these times, when human rights are a prime political, social, religious and ethical issue, no right can exist simply for its own sake.

Some of a parent's rights to custody have been preserved, but not many. A parent still has the right to custody, *unless* the best interests of the child are not served. If divorce, death, or separation has dissolved the family unit, a stranger may be given the custody of a child (Clark, 1968).

But, even if a parent is not a very skillful parent, the state will not interfere with their efforts unless the child is so seriously in trouble as to be within the statutes defining neglected, abused, or delinquent children. Even then the parents may retain custody under some type of state supervision (Clark, 1968).

Custodial rights may be terminated by the state for several reasons beyond the voluntary relinquishment of them. States differ in this regard but in general these are the conditions for the termination: abandonment, neglect or abuse; failure to support; extreme and repeated cruelty; conviction for a felony and the imprisonment thereof; habitual drunkenness or drug addiction; and open and notorious adultery or fornication (Clark, 1968).

In the case of mental illness, if a parent has been judged incompetent, his parental rights, along with other of his rights, are removed, but this condition may be temporary or subject to other specifications. Race and the financial condition of a parent are not counted as factors in termination of rights.

On the positive side of this issue, factors which affect a child remaining within his parents' custody include: the strength and sincerity of the parents' desire for custody, the ability to care for the child as revealed by past performance, the willingness of a new step-parent to care for a child, the physical conditions in which a child will live, and the mental health of the parents.

And so we come to the end of this long and tortuous journey through history. The progress of civilization has changed the matter of parental rights dramatically—from absolute to almost none at all.

Do parents have any rights left? A very few and conditional ones at that. Why has this occurred? I venture to say that, as the issue of human rights in the past two decades has risen to such prominence, and as parents have not demonstrated on the whole that they can legislate themselves, the State has assumed the role of moderator, protector and educator. The rights are gone but the responsibilities remain.

What will be in the offing for parents of the next decade? It is anyone's guess! Mine might be that less government interference in family affairs will be called for. This cry has been heard across the board in recent years and parents, sick of having their efforts and privileges stipulated by a state court, may well begin to defend against further interference.

ED. NOTE: Despite the somewhat pessimistic tone of the author concerning a perceived diminution in the rights of parents vis a vis their children, the rights of parents to parent has been reaffirmed by the United States Supreme Court in recent years. The right to conceive and raise children, the right to have the custody of those children, the right to educate children as one chooses, and the right to be let alone in the private realm of family life are among the fundamental rights protected by the due process and equal protection clauses of the United States Constitution. See *Stanley v. Illinois*, 405 U.S. 645 (1972) and *Lassiter v. Dept. of Social Services*, 452 U.S. 18 (1981). The *Stanley v. Illinois* court noted that "the parent's interest in the companionship, care, custody, and management of his or her children

REFERENCES

Abbott, G. The Child and the State, Volume 1. Chicago: University of Chicago Press, 1938.

Blackston, W. *Commentaries on the Laws of England in Four Books.* London: Robert Bell, Editory, 1765.

Clark, H. *The Law of Domestic Relations.* St. Paul MN: Hornbook Series, 1968.

Diamond, A. *Primitive Law.* London: Watts and Company, 1935.

Driver, G. & Miles, J. *Babylonian Law.* Oxford: Clarendon Press, 1952.

Foster, H., Jr. *A Bill of Rights for Children.* Springfield IL: C.C. Thomas, 1974.

Goldstein, J., Freud, A., Solnit, A. *Beyond the Best Interests of the Child.* NY: Free Press, 1979.

Houlgate, L. *The Child and The State.* Baltimore: Johns Hopkins University Press, 1980.

Kent, J. *Commentaries on American Law*, Volume 2. Boston: Little/ Brown, 1884.

Katz, S. & Inker, M. *Fathers, Husbands, Lovers.* American Bar Association, 1979.

Nicholas, B. *Introduction to Roman Law.* Oxford: Oxford Press, 1962.

Old Testament, King James Version. Oxford: Oxford-Clarendon Press, 1611.

---

is an interest which deserves greater protection than many other personal interests. *Id.* at 641. The Supreme Court also has "little doubt that the Due Process Clause would be offended "[i]f a State were to attempt to force the breakup of a natural family, over the objections of the parents and their children *without some showing of unfitness and for the sole reason that to do so was thought to be in the children's best interest.'* " *Quilloin v. Walcott,* 434 U.S. 245, 266 (1978), quoting from *Smith v. Organization of Foster Families,* 431 U.S. 816, 862-863 (1977). The Supreme Court has also declared that before a state may sever completely and irrevocably the rights of parents in their natural child, due process requires the state support its allegations of unfitness by at least "clear and convincing evidence." Therefore a mere preponderance of the evidence standard, the usual test in civil trials, denies the parent due process. *Santosky v. Krammer,* 455 U.S. 745 (1982). The reader will also note these constitutional principles are applicable not only to the parents of legitimate children, but also to the parents, especially fathers, of illegitimate children. Indeed the Uniform Parentage Act (9A U.L.A. 1) makes no distinction between whether the parents of a child are married or not. The child has a father and a mother without regard to their marital status, and this frees the child of the disabilities associated with being labeled "illegitimate" or given the epithet "bastard."

Schacht, J. *Introduction to Islamic Law,* Oxford: Oxford-Clarendon Press, 1964.

Schwitzgebel, R. & Schwitzgebel, R. *Law and Psychological Practice.* NY: Wiley, 1980.

Walters, D. *Physical and Sexual Abuse of Children: Causes Causes and Treatment.* Bloomington IN: Indiana Press, 1975.

Wilkerson, A. *The Rights of Children: Emergent Concepts of Law and Society.* Philadelphia: Temple University Press, 1973.

Counselor/Therapists and Ethical Decisions Made in Ambiguous Situations

CHAPTER 2

CHARLES A. EATON

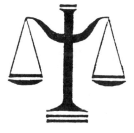

COUNSELOR/ THERAPISTS AND ETHICAL DECISIONS MADE IN AMBIGUOUS SITUATIONS

2

Charles A. Eaton

Familiarity with ambiguous or borderline ethical problems and the ability to assist clients in dealing with them is an essential characteristic of the effective counselor or therapist. The importance of the area of ethical concerns arises from the fact that although individuals may cope adequately with minor value conflicts in daily living, they sooner or later encounter conflicts of value for which they have not been prepared. At such a time, as when the ideals of justice and commitment clash at the point of marital infidelity, individuals may adopt new value perspectives, reorder their hierarchy of values, or perhaps do nothing. It is frequently the case that a prolonged value challenge will result in such personal pain and discomfort that the individual will seek professional aid. Counselors who are unfamiliar with ethical concerns as they relate to the specific world views of their clients will be at a decided disadvantage in assisting them with their crises in values.

The Nature of Ethical Decision Processes

Ethics is properly the study of human values (Adler & Cain, 1962). When these values are viewed as the standard of conduct an individual has constructed to meet various life situations, they are often called moral principles. Moral principles can also be viewed as that body of duties and obligations which a society requires of its members, but for the purposes of this chapter, human values and moral principles will be considered as synonymous, while their exploration, analysis, and clarification will be seen as the province of ethics.

The Current State of Ethics

If ethics is the study of human values, and if all human interests and activities at some point concern values, then it would follow that the study of ethics would be a highly honored portion of every discipline. It is not. Perhaps a confusion exists between the study of ethics and the act of moralizing. If this is true, the fault partly lies with ethicists themselves. If ethics were to be limited to the study of human values, then its utility would rest in the fact that such analysis had cleared the moral landscape from confusing obstacles and rendered the alternatives so clearly that those presented with the necessity of making value decisions could do so responsibly.

However, the ethical endeavor has classicly been tempted (and asked) to do more than clarify the issues. It has been asked for advice, and given it. When this happens, ethics is no longer a study but is a prescriptive and proscriptive activity of moralizing, of inculcating moral values from one group or generation or individual to another. Some would hold that this transmission of values is the central task of culture, while others would view it as a meddling imposition, a tyranny of values. The interpretation of ethics as the transmission, rather than the study, of human values results in the attitude that ethics declares that which we must, ought, and should do. That this attitude is held even by respected ethicists is evident from the preface to the Encyclopedia Brittanica's "Great Ideas" book, *Ethics: The Study of Moral Values*, wherein William Ernest Hocking declared that "ethics is an attempt to make a science of what is in reality an art, the art of right living. . . . .[asking]. . . Can there be a strict science of duty, of the distinction between right and wrong, of the 'You ought?' " (Adler & Cain, 1962, p.v). In answering that question, the story was related of the professor of ethics who began to wonder whether or not his teaching was effective. During a midterm examination the professor put that question to the class and asked for their candid response. One bright student confessed that the teaching of ethics had not noticeably affected his life and that, in the nature of the case, it could not have because:

You cannot *prove* that a man ought to love his neighbor; and if you could, that proof would *not in the least* help him to do so (Adler & Cain, 1962, p. vi).

Ethics as value analysis. We shall have opportunity shortly to see examples of appropriate value communication, but the philosophy student was quite correct in his assessment of ethics as moral advice. It is true that all examinations of human behavior will find at some point a cluster of values, a moral base, even if repugnant to the value perspective of the oberver, which can be viewed as an ethical system. Moreover, this system can be evaluated in terms of its effectiveness in enhancing the life of societies and of individuals within their "being-in-the-world." The consequence of this evaluation and analysis (the proper function of ethics) may very well be a zeal on the part of some to teach, instruct, convert, or forcibly change others, an observable moralizing function. In order to keep a sharp distinction between the analytical and prescriptive interpretations of ethics, there are some who eschew the use of the word "ethics."

Values Clarification. The work of Sidney Simon, Leland Howe, Howard Kirschenbaum, and others, is particularly striking in that it carries out the task of ethics, the study of moral values, with never a reference to either ethics or morals! That the material being studied by these researchers is, in fact, the same value matrix examined by the self-affirming ethicists is evident from the type of questions raised by Simon's 1972 book, *Values Clarification.*

Should Bill and I live together before marriage? Shouldn't we know if we're really compatible?

School seems so irrelevant. Why not drop out and get a better education on my own?

How do I know whether marijuana is really harmful to me or not?

Does religion have some meaning in my life, or is it nothing more than a series of outmoded traditions and customs?

How can I really enjoy working and living and avoid getting into the rat race for the convertible and the house in the suburbs?

What can I do to help improve race relations these days?

Why is it that at the end of every weekend I feel anxious and guilty about all I didn't do? (Simon, Howe & Kirschenbaum, 1972, p. 16)

Values clarification appears to be the method and practice of ethical reflection without visible foundational principles to support the task. Much of this clearly is part of an intent to avoid the moralizing prejudice ascribed to much ethical tradition, while the writers also intend to focus not so much on value/choice possibilities as on the opening up of the moral foundations and principles held by persons taking these exercises. That such conclusions are warranted can be demonstrated by the writing of Sidney Simon himself.

> Moralizing is the direct, although sometimes subtle, inculcation of the adult's values upon the young. The assumption behind moralizing runs something like this: My experience has taught me a certain set of values which I believe would be right for you. Therefore, to save you the pain of coming to these values on your own, and to avoid the risk of your choosing less desirable values, I will effectively transfer my own values to you. . . . Unlike other theoretical approaches to values, [we are] not concerned with the *content* of people's values, but the *process of valuing*. . . . Thus, the values-clarification approach does not aim to instill any particular set of values. Rather the goal. . . is to apply these valuing processes to already formed beliefs and behavior patterns and to those still emerging (Simon, Howe, & Kirschenbaum, 1972, p. 16).

In the above passage, Simon's bias against moralizing is clear, and the implied value base propelling him to design these cryptoethical exercises is that, if not the Socratic belief that the unexamined life is not worth living, at least that the examined life is likely to be healthier, happier, and more fulfilled.

The principles of values-clarification are attractive to therapists of various theoretical orientations. For those who are somewhat directive, it offers techniques of direct and guided reality probing. For more non-directive therapists, the fact that specific values are not suggested or forced upon the client makes this a satisfying technique.

Conflict of Value Constellations or World-views. However, there are certain ethical concerns which truly cry out for a more direct communication of values by a therapist who is sensitive not only to the value system of the client but is also aware of the challenge of other systems. In our pluralistic society, it is inevitable that persons with various values should clash or find themselves inadequate to adjust to changing situations. One example of how an awareness of various value possibilities can aid a therapist can be seen in the example of abortion.

Abortion: Case Example of Ambiguity

That abortion is a chronic "borderline" value issue tangled with ambiguity can be seen by the bafflement of women who at one and the same time affirm that abortion is both a sin and a woman's prerogative ("right"). They would not personally ever consider abortion for themselves but would support the option for other women, yet they believe that the unborn have rights to life—unless the mother has been raped or the pregnancy is the consequence of incest (Yankelovich, Kelly, & White, 1981). It is this type of ethical conundrum which can become personally overwhelming, and which may bring a person to seek professional aid in resolving the conflict. At this point, clarity about the value matrix of the client and of the societal messages on the issue become of immense importance to the therapist. What are the issues involved? The person seeking help has reasons to seek an abortion but is constrained by a value-system which does not allow the taking of life.

Almost desperately the woman attempts to determine what life is, when it begins, and when this developing fetus can claim its independent right to life. The arguments are well known, and the bankruptcy of this line of thinking is evident in the total impasse which has resulted. The reasons for the poverty of this way of looking at abortion, and the consequent anguish of the woman with an unwanted pregnancy, lie in the fact that human life is involved in a continuum.

On the one hand, one could effectively claim that the inevitable directionality of the fertilized ovum means that human life is involved from conception. But, along this continuum, one might also claim, an extreme yet tenable position, that the existence of the ovum is potential human life, lacking only contact with sperm, just as the fetus is potential human life lacking only developmental time. This position is held, by the way, by some who on this basis decry the IUD inasmuch as it interferes with "potential" human life.

On the other hand, one could equally well claim that human life is not attained simply by birth. That is, that human life is not possible outside of the context of a nurturing human culture. In other words, the birth of a human child does not guarantee that it will become "human" unless there is a societal matrix to receive it. If, to continue in this second extreme, all human beings were to be annihilated save for one infant fed by a computer system, would that developing organism be "human?" Surely it is clear that this line of ethical analysis is, has been, and most likely shall be fruitless. Are these options.?

Let us imagine for the moment that the distressed woman is Jewish and that the therapist is aware of her background and of the traditions of Torah. I am aware that at this point we are about to discuss basic principles which might be applied to a particular case, which is casuistry, but we can run that risk as long as it is clear that every value conflict is unique, and must be faced in the context of its uniqueness.

In the Mishna (rabbinic interpretation of Torah), it is affirmed that the community has claims upon every member of the society and responsibilities to every member but that these relationships begin only upon birth. Before birth, the claims and responsibilities are those of the mother. This is not different in concept from traditional laws regarding certain types of property. For example, a fish in a lake is public property of the community until it is caught by a duly licensed individual, at which point it becomes private property. In a reverse sense, the unborn child is the "property" of its mother until birth, at which time it is jointly and unequally claimed by the mother, family, and state. Such a perspective and ethical content does not give insight into a particular therapeutic process, but it does provide for the therapist an alternate value base from which to assist the client in her options, where her former perspective placed her in the intolerable position of choosing either for murder or a desperately unwanted birth.

For the moment, continue to look at the example of abortion, this time assuming that the person is inclined toward a Christian perspective. At this point the therapist would be quite clear that there is no Biblical reference to "rights" of unborn children. More importantly, there is no reference to rights of any kind at all for anyone. The deep concern in the Bible toward aid to widows, orphans, the poor, sick, imprisoned, etc., is not based upon their "right" to that compassion but upon our *responsibility* to be merciful. The concept of Human Rights, by the way, is a modern consequence of French rationalism, a theory of natural rights held by Marsilius of Padua, John Locke, Jean Jacques Rousseau, and others, which forms the basis of our Declaration of Independence.

> We hold these truths to be self-evident, that all men are created equal, that they are endowed by their Creator with certain inalienable Rights, that among these are Life, Liberty, and the pursuit of Happiness... (Declaration of Independence).

The Philosophy of Rationalism

Where do we get the idea that "inalienable Rights" are an endowment given to us by our Creator? The source is not found in any religion at all, but in the philosophy of Rationalism. This is not to quibble with the practical utility of the idea, but to be quite definite in asserting that there are other categories available to various value traditions. The Christian tradition contains several options (others will be discussed later), but at this point the countering of "responsibilities" for "rights" is most appropriate. If we raise the question of responsibility we can ask what the responsibility of the community is toward the unborn fetus. Does it include the nurture, education, and support of the mother? If so, what is the ratio of shared responsibility between society and the individual mother? If she has the greater responsibility prior to birth, does it include the responsibility for judgment as to termination of pregnancy? In an ambiguous area, does society allow the mother to do something which is appropriate in her eyes and wrong in the eyes of society? Such questions, again, are not in themselves therapeutic devices, but they stem from an awareness of options which would enable a therapist to counter the sense of impasse by the presentation of alternate ways of viewing abortion.

That an understanding of the values held by a client and an awareness of reasonable adjustments within that matrix is crucially important for an effective therapist can be dramatically seen in the encounter of Viktor Frankl, a survivor of Auschwitz, with a rabbi who also had been in the death camp of Auschwitz and whose wife and six children had been killed there. The rabbi had come to Frankl for counsel; his presenting complaint was his distress that his second wife was sterile. Frankl observed that life without procreation is not meaningless. For, if life itself were meaningless, it could not be made meaningful simply by its perpetuation. The rabbi clearly was not having his central needs met, and, after further dialogue, he said that he despaired because there would be no child to say the Prayer of the Dead (Kaddish) for him. When Frankl countered that he would still see his children in the life to come, the rabbi broke into bitter tears saying that he would never see his children since they had died as martyrs (*L'kiddush hashem*, For the santification of God's name") and would occupy the highest places in heaven, whereas he, a sinful old man, knew well that none of the innocent survived the death-camps and he therefore could not see them for all eternity. A completely secular therapist would, at this point, have great difficulty dealing with values which had been held over a long period of time and had gone through the testing by fire of concentration camps. A Christian counselor might be tempted to speak of reconciliation and redemption in Jesus Christ, but the likelihood is that these value images would be too far from the world-view of the rabbi. And so Viktor Frankl stayed within the rabbinical tradition, and said:

> Is it not conceivable, Rabbi, that precisely this was the meaning of your surviving your children; that you may be purified through these years of suffering, so that finally you, too, though not innocent like your children, may *become* worthy of joining them in Heaven? Is it not written in the Psalms that God preserves all your tears? So perhaps your sufferings were not in vain (Frankl, 1967, pp. 85-87).

The rabbi now could interpret his own sorrow as having had a cleansing effect upon his own soul, and he felt relief for the first time in years. Such a therapeutic conclusion could only have happened in a situation where the therapist was aware of the values held by the client. Does this mean that the therapist/client relationship must always be one of value correspondence or, at the least, of an understanding on the part of the therapist of the context of the value conflict? Not always. It would, of course, be desirable for the therapist to understand the world-view of the client but there are examples of successful exceptions.

For example, allow me to cite a case of modern exorcism. A white, Anglo-Saxon, Freudian psychoanalyst happened to be practicing medicine and psychiatry among a group of American Indians in Oregon, when he was presented with a girl who seemed troubled by factors uniquely related to the value system of her world-view. During the day she attended an integrated school in a small town, and was dressed in every way like the other children. After school she returned home, assumed native garb, and braided her hair in the style of her village. She was aware at this time that her grandfather had been the shaman (medicine-man) of the village, and that he had specifically bequeathed to her the role of becoming the next shaman. It is true that inheritance of function is usually considered an aspect of priesthood which distinguishes priests from shamans, but apparently some shamans are elected, while some priests surely are "called."

The precipitating crisis which brought her to the psychoanalyst was that during a girls' summer camp experience, several girls went at night to an old and abandoned house which was said to have been haunted. There was the usual thrill of breaking camp rules to which was added the special spice of a mysterious and forbidden spirit-abode. Upon returning to her village, the girl was terrified by visions of blood which covered every part of the floor of her home. After suffering with these visions for some time, the girl was brought to the psychoanalyst. His conversations with the mother and daughter revealed that severe conflicts were occurring on the level of deeply held values, values with which he was unfamiliar. So, showing immense good sense, the doctor asked the mother, "What do you do in situations like this?"

She replied that persons were exorcized. He then asked if that could be done, and if, at the same time, her daughter might be exempted from becoming the next shaman for the village. The answer to both questions was in the affirmative, the mother stating that the requirements were that a certain number of women of the village make specific preparations and then hold a service of dance and song over a period of several days. The psychiatrist then asked them to report back, and the consequence was that the girl was relieved both of her bloody visions and psychological distress. In this case, the sensitivity of the therapist to value conflicts, even though quite foreign and unknown to him, was the most significant element in final success (Cox, 1973).

Principles of Professional Strategy

If the therapist comes to the conviction that an ethical analysis of underlying values is essential for effective therapy, that analysis can then be achieved in a number of ways, for all theories of therapy contain techniques appropriate to their theory. Frequently the conflict of values is clear and evident. In such situations, the task is not so much to discover the nature of the conflict as it is to see what in the client's value world-view provides inhibitions or openness to value reorientation. For example, when Viktor Frankl's first wife was separated from him and was to be sent to a concentration camp for women, he said to her, "Do anything to live (Thielicke, 1966, p. 24)."

His reason for saying this was that he knew that her value system held high esteem for marital fidelity. He also knew that in the face of death some women had gained life by becoming camp prostitutes for the SS officers. What he was saying was that she should reorder the hierarchy of her values so that survival would be given the top priority. [She did not live.]

There are times when an arrangement of moral values which has been useful in the past no longer meets the needs of the present. At this point, the task of the therapist is to clarify the issues in such a way that the client may make effective decisions. This is not at all to say that the therapist is to give advice. The ethical process is not the instruction of what a person is obliged to do; strictly speaking, it is the exploration of the possibilities of what we may do if we decide to.

However, it is not the intent of this chapter to discuss the various end-points of classical systems of philosophical ethics; the intent is rather to understand how values-analysis is appropriate to the therapeutic process. In doing this, the therapist must be aware that not all value systems are asking the same questions; therefore the *direction* of the therapist's value-thinking may be different from that of the client. For example, the therapist might be such a doctrinaire Kantian as to believe that there is only one legitimate impulse to action, namely, to act in such a way that "the maxims of this action" can be made the "principle of universal legislation." Such a perspective would have specific consequences for therapy, as would any other ethical perspective.

But let us instead imagine that the therapist is dedicated to working within clients' world-views while temporarily suspending the therapist's own view. If this were possible in practice, the therapist would still have to become aware of the cultural matrix of clients' value-systems and the various therapeutic tactics available within a particular tradition. In doing this, the therapist would discover a multitude of ethical categories. Among these would be the earnest search for that which is right, true, just, or good. These are the classic categories of Western ethical thinking, but there is another equally important category found in several traditions; that ethical thinking simply put is this: "What is the will of God?"

Some secular therapists might be tempted to refer the client to a member of the clergy at that point, but that may not be necessary. What is necessary is to know something about ethical questions which are seen from the perspective of a religious tradition.

Resolution of Ethical Problems in Protestantism and Catholicism

From a Protestant perspective, the uniquely "Christian" element in ethics is to be found exclusively in the motivation of an action. In the famous polemic of Jesus against the Pharisees the point is driven home repeatedly that outward actions and deeds, regardless of how noble, beneficial, and good, are worthless if there is not an appropriate inward motive. This perspective is developed in Matthew in a series of "woes."

> Woe to you, scribes and Pharisees, hypocrites! for you are like whitewashed tombs, which outwardly appear beautiful, but within they are full of dead men's bones and all uncleanness. So you also appear righteous to men, but within you are full of hypocrisy and iniquity (Matthew 23:27,28).

This inward motive is to be an impulse toward love of God and neighbor which is to spring from the center of a person's being.

> Whatever you do, do it from the heart (*ex psyche*), as to the Lord, and not to men (Colossian 3:23).

The client, in struggling with the question of the will of God in a particular situation, will seek answers in one of three ways: appeal to the authority of scriptures, guidance from ecclesiastical tradition or leadership, direct prayer. What the therapist needs to be clear about is that the only means available to know the ultimate divine will are all ambiguous and uncertain. Consequently, the history of religious response to ethical problems has not sought certainty of revelation. Instead, it has placed the focus upon the attitude and motivations of the believer. A convenient summary of this perspective is found in the writing of Reformed theologian Helmut Thielicke:

> Love alone does justice to the true intention of the Law, which is to bring about a conformity with the will of God. He who loves finds that he is in agreement with the one who is the object of his love. Hence an action done in love is an action performed out of conformity. But this action cannot be casuistically predetermined by laws. Because it is the objectification and expression of the love which motivates it, it has the freedom to take any of the most varied forms. This is what Augustine meant with his famous dictum, "Love, and do what you want" (*Dilige et fac quod vis*). The commandment of love is thus the end of casuistry. It is what empowers to freedom (Thielicke, 1966, p. 24).

These principles may be, from a Protestant perspective, "the end of casuistry," but they mark the foundation of a new Roman Catholic casuistry. This most recent attempt at ethical guidance in the Catholic church can be seen in the book, *Human Sexuality: New Directions in American Catholic Thought* (Kosnick, 1977). If classic casuistry (which means the "study of cases") attempted to define moral principles which could be applied in specific situations, the new directions of Catholic thought are new indeed.

Commissioned by The Catholic Theological Society in America, this study combines historical, theological, behavioral, and practical concerns in an attempt "to bring Christian theological reflection to bear on the complex phenomenon of human sexuality in the hope of providing some helpful pastoral guidance to beleagured pastors, priests, [and] counselors (Kosnick, 1977, p. xiv)." Their conclusions do not represent current official

Roman Catholic teaching, but do provide a practical guide to directions in which such teaching is moving, and familiarity with this document would heighten the sensitivity of therapists who are unfamiliar with Catholic tradition and practice. Actually, the book is difficult to find, especially in Catholic bookstores, as it was never given the "Imprimatur," and drew the condemnation of Pope John Paul II.

The "new" element in casuistry is that although specific cases are studied, general principles are developed which are based on the "motive" element discussed above. Yet, complain the Catholic scholars, if love of God and neighbor is commended as the basis for an ethically responsible life, we are incomplete in our responsibility toward people if we do not assist them in seeing the implications of certain types of behavior and of finding motivation for certain other styles of behavior. The shocking element of the new studies is that they moved decisively and swiftly away from the old position that one can know what is right or wrong about moral choices in general and thereby order one's life accordingly. They were also not willing to accept as an alternative a completely relative and subjective attitude toward ethical reflection and moral action. They recognized the importance of the personal element as indispensable in the ethical process, but they were aware that it could easily neglect the "social and communal" implications of sexual behavior. The writer's operating principles included the following:

A sound approach to the moral evaluation of sexual behavior must do justice to several extremely complex factors:

(1) It must recognize both the objective and the subjective aspects of human behavior as indispensable to any genuine moral judgment. To ignore either aspect results either in a rigid moral externalism or self-serving moral subjectivism.

(2) It must acknowledge the radical complexity and unity of the human person's sexual nature and avoid any attempt to establish a hierarchy of creativity over integration or vice-versa.

(3) It must demand a constant awareness of the delicate, interpersonal dimension of this experience which constitutes an integral part of any moral standard or judgment (Kosnick, 1977, p. 90).

As a consequence, the writers attacked the ancient, simple, and direct question, "Is this act moral or immoral?" (which is the underlying question in many ethical questions) as being highly flawed in two significant ways. In the first place, such simple questions do a "disservice to the complexity of the human moral enterprise" (Kosnick, 1977, p. 91). They suggested that ethically responsible acts can happen without the components of human decision and intention, and that the process of ethical reflection can take place in this vacuum. But, say the writers, judgments regarding human sexuality must include not only the specific and observable phenomenon but also the context and intention. But there are other reasons to indicate that the old simple questions—and answers—were flawed.

> [They imply] a greatly oversimplified understanding of sexuality. That any specific act can be measured and evaluated in a way totally adequate to the intricate manifold of human experience is dubious at best. Human sexuality is simply too complex, too mysterious, too sacred a human experience for such categorization. Tentativity is inevitable in the attempt to discern the objective significance of such a mysterious and many splendored reality" (Kosnick, 1977, p. 91).

Yet the author did not feel stymied in the task of giving ethical guidance. Refusing to settle for one principle of "love" as is typical of much Protestant "Situation Ethics," the conclusion was made that it would be possible to design a values-grid whose use would assist a person in applying personal, social, and religious principles in the uniqueness of a specific situation, without drawing conclusions for others. Among those values which they felt were particularly conducive to health and growth within the human community, were the following:

Positive Human sexuality is likely to be:
  (1) Self-liberating
  (2) Other-Enriching
  (3) Honest
  (4) Faithful
  (5) Socially responsible
  (6) Life-serving
  (7) Joyous

Where such qualities prevail, one can be reasonably sure that the sexual behavior that has brought them forth is wholesome and moral. On the contrary, where sexual conduct becomes personally frustrating and self-destructive, manipulative and enslaving of others, deceitful and dishonest, inconsistent and unstable, indiscriminate and promiscuous, irresponsible and non-life-serving, burdensome and repugnant, ungenerous and un-Christlike, it is clear the God's ingenious gift for calling us to creative and integrative growth has been seriously abused (Kosnick, 1977, p. 95).

Even a casual glance at the above positive and negative value-grids reveals the revolutionary nature of this document, for whereas Catholics at one time could unequivocably declare that marriage is good and homosexual relations were evil, now all conditions of sexual communication are seen to be subject to the same value-grid and may fail or succeed in any specific situation. Categorical generalization has had its day, but individual behavior is subject to and aided by a simple, but complex, value-grid. The main body of Kosnick's book, by the way, consists of pastoral guidelines to parish priests as they assist persons who find themselves in ambiguous or borderline ethical questions related to specific sexual behavior possibilities. It perhaps does not need to be noted that a value-grid which is useful in one ambiguous area is helpful in others as well.

In conclusion, then, the counselor/therapist is likely to find that clients not only have problems in living, but also have problems in relating their actions to their value systems. Whereas each theory of therapy has tools for uncovering and dealing with such value conflicts, it has been the position of this paper that the therapist is most likely to be effective in using these tools when the full picture of the client's world-view is known, as well as those alternative perspectives which allow for new interpretation and decision from within the general context of the client's value system.

REFERENCES

Adler, M. & Cain, S. *The Great Ideas Program (Vol. 8): Ethics: The Study of Moral Values*. Chicago: Encyclopedia Brittanica, Inc., 1962.

Cox, R. (Ed.) *Religious Systems and Psychotherapy.* Springfield Il: C.C. Thomas, 1973.

Frankl, V. *Psychotherapy and Existentialism.* NY: Simon & Schuster, 1967.

Kosnick, A., et al. *Human Sexuality: New Directions in American Catholic Thought.* NY: Paulist Press, 1977.

Simon, S., Howe, L., & Kirschenbaum, H. *Values Clarification: A Handbook of Practical Strategies for Teachers and Students.* NY: Hart Publishing Co., 1972.

Thielicke, Helmut. *Theological Ethics (Vol. I): Foundations.* Philadelphia: Fortress Press, 1966.

Yankelovich, Skelly, & White. Abortion: Women speak out. In *Life Magazine*, November 1981, 45–54.

The Rights of Children

CHAPTER 3

NANCY G. SCHUELLER

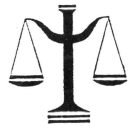

THE RIGHTS OF CHILDREN

3

Nancy G. Schueller

In the Massachusetts Bay Colony it was a law that "...if any child or children above sixteen years old, and of sufficient understanding shall curse or smite their natural father or mother, he or they shall be put to death" (Beyer, 1977, p. 84). Throughout the 1700s and up into the late 1800s the predominant view of children was that they were innately sinful and only potentially redeemable through the constant and concerted efforts of the parents. There was no thought of "children's rights."

It is noteworthy that a society for the prevention of cruelty to children was organized in 1874 in New York, ten years *after* the establishment of a society for the prevention of cruelty to animals!

In modern times, there are child advocates, those who try to help children and prevent them from being abused or neglected. Child advocates work with or against those systems which affect children deleteriously. One major advocacy organization is the Children's Defense Fund (CDF). The CDF challenges harmful practices to children through court action (Gross & Gross, 1977).

The courts have traditionally seen parents as having a "natural right" to decide what is best for their children and have usually tried not to interfere with parental rights and family privacy. However, recent legislation and judicial decisions have reduced parental power in a number of areas.

For example, minor children living away from their parents can now obtain medical treatment on their own. Also, children twelve years of age and over, even if still living at home can independently obtain help for venereal disease, birth control and substance abuse (Beyer, 1977).

A number of court cases will illustrate the changes which have taken place over the past few years. In *In re Gault* (1976) the Supreme Court decided that the Fourteenth Amendment and the Bill of Rights also apply to children. *Tinker v. Des Moines School District* (1969) declared that under the constitution, children are "persons." But this has still not meant that children legally have all the same rights as adults. *Planned Parenthood v. Danforth* (1976) held that adolescents under eighteen years of age may obtain an abortion without having parental consent.

Thus minors do have rights that are protected by the Constitution. Some children under the age of eighteen become emancipated minors and are free from parental control through marriage or independent living. Today minors can even sue their parents (Beyer, 1977; Stier, 1978). Yet some advertising has been outlawed because it could unduly influence children who are not old enough to decide for themselves what they need or should use. The issue here is the age of the children involved. Children are not miniature adults. Perhaps children should be granted rights the same as adults, but dependent upon their emotional and intellectural development, along the lines of Piaget's intellectual stages.

For example, children would be given more rights when they reached the stage of formal operations, as opposed to concrete operations (Baumrind, 1978). Of course, if one follows this train of thought far enough it has the unpleasant hint that adults who are declared emotionally or intellectually immature could have some of their rights taken away. This already does happen if adults are seriously intellectually impaired and declared incompetent by the courts, but it does not happen for immaturity alone.

Parental autonomy, children's rights, and state concerns must all be considered and balanced. A summary of recent case law suggests that:

- Children are persons and enjoy constitutional rights and protections.
- Children's interests have generally been seen as allied with those of their parents.
- In conflicts between the interests of parents and children, the rights of children and the role of the state are still without clear delineation.

● The state may act to limit parents' discretion with regard to their child. When it does, its interests are twofold: (a) protecting the interest of the child, and (b) furthering general societal interests in the well-being of its youth (Ellis, 1974, pp. 875-876).

Serena Stier (1978) has proposed that legislation should be more active. Currently legislation waits for the results of judicial decision. However this process is usually better at striking down existing laws rather than creating beneficial and protective laws for children. It also tends to be overly individualized and often does not resolve the issues involved.

"Legislatively, however, there has been a liberalizing trend in evaluating the capacity of a minor to make adult decisions which is expressed in terms of a 'mature minor rule' " (Stier, 1978, p. 52). Feshback and Feshback (1978, p. 168) have proposed that ". . .how a parent rears a child should be an open matter, available for discussion, help and inquiry." They argued that the welfare of the child is reason to invade family privacy although care should be taken to leave family boundaries intact.

Professionals who are involved with children could be given the right to inquire of the parents as to how they are disciplining the children, etc., and expect that the parent will respond to the questions. The professionals could then offer information and alternative child rearing procedures, if appropriate and warranted. Their purpose would be to support and educate parents. This would not be a legal procedure but a social pressure. Custom and law say that the family is the main socializing agent in the lives of children, but the state and society do have an interest in the welfare and rights of children. Children are no longer considered to be possessions and they are certainly not slaves of the parents.

Berlin (1975) has proposed the following Bill of Rights for Children which is derived in part from the rights developed by the Joint Commission on Mental Health for Children:

BILL OF RIGHTS

We hold these truths inalienable for all children:

(1) The Right to be born wanted.
(2) The Right to be born healthy.
(3) The Right to live in a healthful environment.
(4) The right to live in a family whose basic economic needs are met.

(5) The Right to continuous and loving care both at home and in school.
(6) The Right to acquire intellectual and emotional skills for effective citizenship.
    a . The Right to dignity in school.
    b.   The Right to humane and concerned treatment under the Law and by Courts.
    c.   The Right to child-centered divorce and custody laws.
(7) The Right to meaningful employment.
(8) The Right to diagnostic, treatment, and rehabilitative care through facilities which are appropriate to children's special needs and which keep them as closely as possible within their normal social setting.
(9) The Right to racial and ethnic identity, self-determination, and a real and functional equality of opportunity to the above rights.
(10) The Right to political participation through education for informed citizenship (Berlin, 1975, p. 5).

Berlin wrote the above list of rights to help point out the great inequalities between children and adults in our society. He believed that it was necessary for our survival that these rights be granted to children.

Gerald P. Koocher (1976) pointed out that the day-to-day activities of mental health professionals often violates the individual rights of children. These rights are not guaranteed privileges by law but are moral and ethical considerations. Actually, the right to mental health treatment has not yet been extended to children. The right to refuse treatment is similarly enigmatic. In the past, there were two ways for a child to be placed in a residential treatment facility, placement by the parents or by the juvenile courts. Previously parents could place children in institutions for the mentally ill or retarded without any sort of review and over the protests of the children. This parental right was sometimes abused by parents who merely wished someone else to care for their troublesome children (Miller & Burt, 1977; Beyer, 1977).

Saville v. Treadway (1974) held that (at least in Tennessee) all admissions of minors under sixteen years to a facility for the retarded must be reviewed by an independent board. In Pennsylvania (1975), *Bartley v. Kremens* declared that when a child is admitted to a mental health facility, a preliminary court hearing must be held within three days and a full hearing held within two weeks to determine if the placement is appropriate.

New regulations state that adolescents who protest their commitment may obtain a court review and be represented by an appointed attorney. The courts can place adolescents only if they are a danger to themselves or others. Some states have regulated that all children who are committed have a right to an appointed attorney.

Adolescents can refuse or leave an inpatient facility at the age of sixteen unless they meet the criteria for adult commitment. At thirteen years, they may request court hearings to protest commitment by their parents and they must be told what their rights are. The *O'Connor v. Donaldson* decision has been extended to adolescents and younger children. This means that civilly committed persons have a right to be released if they are not a danger to themselves or others, can survive in the community with help, and are only receiving custodial care within the institution. The American Psychological Association has proposed that minors twelve years and over be given the same due process protections as adults for commitment (Beyer, 1977; Miller & Burt, 1977; Stier, 1978).

The right of adolescents to challenge inpatient treatment has created some problems. "There is clinical psychiatric evidence that when authority figures implicitly act with children against their parents, the results of treatment are generally unsatisfactory" (Miller and Burt, 1977, p. 153). Children who need treatment the most may be the most verbally opposed to it; for example, adolescents who are already struggling with dependency and autonomy issues.

Many facilities will not accept those children who are involved in court proceedings because they fear it will make treatment more complicated and confusing due to the influence of the children's lawyers and court investigators. Often adolescents confuse being told their rights with being rejected. They get the idea that they are not wanted in treatment. If a court does force a sixteen-year-old to stay in treatment on the basis of the therapist's testimony, the therapeutic relationship may be totally destroyed. If the courts emancipate the sixteen-year-old, then he or she may perceive the therapist as having been "devalued" and thus the therapeutic relationship may be destroyed regardless of the court decision.

The basic issue here seems to be the balance between personal liberty which Constitutionally cannot be denied without due process and the parental rights to make important decisions regarding children, without interference by the state. The courts should carefully scrutinize this issue, especially when treatment may include locked wards, restraints, chemical agents and geographical remoteness. The concept of "least restrictive alternative" is applicable. Those facilities which are the most restrictive should require the most stringent legal proceedings. Some therapists suggest that if an adolescent keeps running away from more open treatment centers, then legal proceedings should be considered, but not before that time. When children are not old enough to speak for themselves, an advocate should be appointed to speak for them.

Children are most often introduced to psychotherapy by their parents. Sometimes a major problem for the therapist is deciding what goals of therapy are best for the child. The goals the parents may request or the goals of the child may not be the same at all. If the child does not want treatment, this problem is further compounded. Many times the difficulties may lie within the family's functioning rather than within the child. The therapist may want to consider family therapy as a viable alternative. If the parents refuse, then the therapist is left with having to decide if he can be a therapeutic agent for this child at all, or if he should decline to take the child as a patient (Koocher, 1976).

Prudent psychotherapists, when deciding the goals of treatment should listen to the parents, use their own professional judgment, be aware of professional literature related to the specific problems involved, the child's assessment of the situation, and the values of the community. The therapist must then strike a balance among the values held by the child, the parents, and those of society. The wishes of young and teen-aged children should be carefully considered but should not be the deciding factor alone.

> ...while it is desirable for the therapist to work in consonance with the child's expressed desires, one need not wait for the child's consent to psychotherapeutic help if the apparent and expressed misery of the child requires direct action to alleviate the present state of discomfort and to

prevent future unhappiness (Rosen, Recker, & Bentler, 1978, p. 127).

Principle 6 from the *Ethical Standards of Psychogists*, regarding the welfare of the consumer, can be applied to this issue of goals for children in therapy. Children are the clients and their welfare is the overriding consideration.

It has been further suggested that children have the results of clinical evaluations discussed with them. It reassures them that the nature of their difficulties is not unspeakable and is an indication to them that they are respected as individuals. Of course, the clinician must only share what is appropriate and capable of being understood by that particular child.

Again the welfare of the child-client is the criterion of all such communications. A thoughtful follow-up discussion of an evaluation can help prepare the children for treatment, clear up misperceptions and reassure them of the plans and goals of treatment. Areas of strengths and special talents should also be included in this discussion. Discussing the results with children can also encourage the parents to respect the individuality and competency of their children. It is unnecessary to give children a diagnosis which could be damaging to their self-esteem and self-concept. But the difficulties the child is experiencing can gently be discussed in terms like fears and worries. Naturally these discussions would be severely limited or not appropriate for extremely young children or those with severe retardation or neurological impairment.

Ross (1974) proposed four basic tenets for the child as a psychotherapy patient:

- Children have the right to be told the truth.
- Children have the right to be treated with respect.
- The child-client has the right to be taken seriously.
- The child has a right to meaningful participation in decision-making that applies to his or her life.

Confidentiality is another major issue regarding children in therapy. The patient is the holder of this privilege. "The privacy of communication with professionals who deal with children is protected by professional ethics and should be maintained with vigilance (Feshback & Feshback, 1978, p. 173).

Historically the psychotherapist-patient privilege is like that of the doctor-patient.

> Since the very essence of psychotherapy is confidential personal revelations about matters the patient is normally reluctant to discuss, any communications to a psycho therapist during the course of consultation are (1) essentially of a confidential and secret nature; (2) less likely and far more difficult to obtain if the patient knows that they may be revealed during the course of some future lawsuit; (3) the outgrowth of a relationship which should be fostered, and (4) the type of information which is revealed would produce far fewer benefits to justice than the consequent injury to the entire field of psychotherapy (*Northwestern University Law Review*, 1952, p. 387).

If a child discloses dangerous or self-destructive plans, the therapist must carefully evaluate the validity of those claims. In that instance, confidentiality may be broken in the best interests of the child but there is a danger that the child's statements may have been a test to see if the therapist could be trusted. If it were a test, then to break confidentiality may destroy the therapeutic relationship (Koocher, 1979; Ross, 1974).

Another instance when confidentiality can be broken is when the patient is under sixteen years and reasonably believed to have been the victim of a crime. For instance, the therapist is mandated to report suspicions of child abuse or neglect. If the child is seen alone, some therapists have suggested that the therapist should have no contact with the parents whatsoever in order to insure confidentiality to the child. Some parents reasonably desire periodic reports on the progress being made in therapy. To do this, the therapist may discuss with the children what they wish to tell the parents and obtain permission from them to do so. A child can also be encouraged by the therapist to share important information with the parents (see ed. note).

Ed. Note: There is mandatory reporting of child abuse in all 50 states, regardless of age. For example, in California, the law states: "...any child care custodian, medical practitioner, nonmedical practitioner, or employee of a child protective agency who has knowledge of or observes a child in his or her professional capacity or within the scope of his or her employment whom he or she knows or reasonably suspects has been the victim of child abuse shall report the known or suspected instance of child abuse to a child protective agency immediately or as soon as practically possible by telephone and shall prepare and send a written report thereof within 36 hours of receiving the information concerning the incident."

Within the issue of record keeping, the rights of the child must again be balanced with the rights of the parents. Parents should not have absolute access when their interests are known to conflict with those of the child. Any child old enough to understand the decision not to allow the parents to view the records, should have the right to make that decision. Children fourteen years and over have access to their own records, except when viewing those records could result in their becoming violent and potentially harmful to themselves or others, or when those records could cause them to become severely depressed.

For the records of younger children, the therapist must assess whether or not letting the parents see the records would create a dangerous situation for the child. It seems wise for the therapist to consider carefully what goes into the records (Brant, Garinger, & Brant, 1976).

The confidentiality of records kept on a child has implications for the researcher. Long-term follow-up studies of child research is now nearly impossible. Evaluations of interventions with disturbed youngsters and control populations virtually cannot be done because many records are now closed to the researcher. For instance, school and birth records are unavailable. The privacy and confidentiality rights of children are of vital importance. Researchers do not desire to violate these rights, but they do need some statistical data contained in these records. The current trend of destroying records and keeping confidential material out of records may mean that future generations are deprived of potentially beneficial knowledge. The issue of confidentiality is not solved by the lack of record keeping or by prohibiting researchers from seeing some kinds of records (Robins, 1977).

A bigger problem for researchers is the issue of "informed consent" and "voluntariness." The use of children in past research has been quite valuable. The rubella and poliomyelitis vaccines were developed mostly through research done on healthy children that undoubtedly could not be done today. Unfortunately there have been past abuses of children in research especially with retarded and orphaned children.

One of the more notorious instances in the 1950s involved healthy retarded children who were injected with hepatitis to test the researcher's cure. This was done on the grounds that hepatitis was rampant in the institution where the children were being placed, and they probably would have gotten hepatitis anyway. Parents were persuaded to give consent, as doing so would vastly speed up the admittance process (Frankle, 1978).

It appears impossible for young children to give informed consent. The U.S. Department of Health, Education and Welfare (HEW) has determined that the age of discretion for children is seven years. For research using children seven years and over, informed consent is necessary, though there is some problem in the variation of individual children's mental age. Parents may give consent by proxy. The APA's Ad Hoc committee on Ethical Standards in Psychological Research (1973) said that ". . .free and informed consent should be obtained from a person whose primary interest is in the participant's welfare" (APA, 1973, pp. 35–36). Sometimes economic and social pressures can influence the parents so that they are not always looking out for the best interests of their child. Also, there is no firm legal basis for parental consent for children involved in non-therapeutic experimentation (Frankle, 1978; Rosen, Reckers, & Bentler, 1978).

It is much easier to use older adolescents as they can give consent for themselves. Even when young children are told that they do not have to participate in research unless they want to and that they can quit at any time, children are used to obeying adults and may find it difficult to refuse to participate or to signal that they wish to terminate their participation (Beyer, 1977; Keith-Spiegel, 1976).

Investigators are responsible for assessing the potential physical risks as well as possible psychological and social harm involved in participation in research. It was suggested by HEW that research should be done on animals and adults first, before being done with children. If it is a controlled experiment, then if the experimental treatment is found to be beneficial, it should be offered to the experimental control group also (Keith-Spiegel, 1976). Risks are only acceptable if the research can be done no other way, and the potential benefit is significant and far outweighs the potential risk (Frankle, 1978).

When the treatment or research has no potential benefit for the participants, then more restrictions are needed. In 1973 HEW proposed that children could participate in biomedical research when the risk of a proposed study was generally considered not significant, and the potential benefit was explicit. The consent of both parents is needed, and children, so far as they can understand, must be given the right to refuse to participate. If there are no parents or adopted parents, the child cannot participate, if there is any risk at all, unless the child is seriously ill and the experimental therapy is the only chance for potential benefit (Beyer, 1977).

Many investigators feel that research should *never* be done with institutionalized children. Others say that proxy consent is appropriate, if (1) it is probable the child would give consent if he could; (2) the danger or discomfort is so remote or minimal that normal individuals would give consent; and (3) there are potential benefits for a great many. Nontherapeutic experimentation with high risks is *never* allowed even with parental consent (Frankle, 1978).

Children have a right to a debriefing after the experiment, just as adults do. The primary objective is to ensure that the child leaves with no undesirable aftermath. The APA has suggested that:

> . . . certain misconceptions should not be removed (for example, if a child was previously led to believe that he performed better than he actually did) or even that additional misconceptions should be induced (the experimenter may try to convince the child that he did better than he actually did) (Keith-Spiegel, 1976, p. 71).

This requirement seems to complicate the issue of debriefing. The researcher must balance between research interests and the welfare of the participants.

Guidelines for research with children require that proposals be examined by the Ethical Review Board at the sponsoring HEW agency and by the Protection Committee at the grantee institution. The proposal should be reviewed by up to three more review boards depending upon the risk factors involved. But, the best protection of children in research and therapy is still found in professional self-control and adherence to ethical standards (Keith-Spiegel, 1976).

REFERENCES

American Psychological Association. *Ethical Standards of Psychologists*, 1979.

Baurind, D. Reciprocal rights and responsibilities in parent-child relations, *Journal of Social Issues*, 1978, *34*(2), 179–106.

Bennett, W. Rights of children, *Family Coordinator*, 1977, *26*(4), 333–337.

Berlin, I. We advocate this Bill of Rights. In I. Berlin (Ed.), *Advocacy for Child Mental Health*, NY: Brunner/Mazel, 1975.

Beyer, H. Changes in the parent-child legal relationship: What they mean to the clinician, *Journal of Autism and Childhood Schizophrenia*, 1977, *7*(1), 84–96.

Brant, J., Garinger, G., & Brant, R. Do you want to see our files on you? In G. Koocher (Ed.), *Children's Rights and the Mental Health Professional*, NY: John Wiley & Sons, 1976.

California Association of Marriage and Family Counselors, *Ethical Standards for Marriage and Family Counselors*, 1978.

Northwestern University Law Review, Confidential communications to a psychotherapist: A new testimonial privilege, 1952, *47*(3), 384–389.

Ellis, J. Volunteering children: parental commitment of minors to mental institutions, *California Law Review*, 1974, *62*, 840–916.

Feshback, S. & Feshback, N. Child advocacy and family privacy, *Journal of Social Issues*, 1978, *34*(2), 168–178.

Frankle, M. Social, legal and political responses to ethical issues in the use of children as experimental subjects, *Journal of Social Issues*, 1978, *34*(2), 101–113.

Gross, B. & Gross, R. *The Children's Rights Movement*, NY: Anchor Press, 1977.

Keith-Spiegel, P. Children's rights as participants in research. In G. Koocher (Ed.), *Children's Rights and the Mental Health Professional*, NY: John Wiley & Sons, 1976.

Koocher, G. An introduction: Why children's rights? In G. Koocher (Ed.), *Children's rights and the Mental Health Professional,* NY: John Wiley & Sons, 1976.

Koocher, G. A Bill of Rights for children in psychotherapy. In G. Koocher (Ed.), *Children's Rights and the Mental Health Professional*, NY: John Wiley & Sons, 1976.

LoCicero, A. The right to know: Telling children the results of clinical evaluation. In G. Koocher (Ed.), *Children's Rights and the Mental Health Professional,* NY: John Wiley & Sons, 1976.

Miller, D. & Burt, R. Children's rights on entering therapeutic institutions, *American Journal of Psychiatry,* 1977, *134*(2), 153–156.

Robins, L. Problems in follow-up studies, *American Journal of Psychiatry,* 1977, *134*(8), 904–907.

Rosen, A., Reckers, G., & Bentler, P. Ethical issues in the treatment of children, *Journal of Social Issues,* 1978, *34*(2), 122–136.

Ross, A. *The rights of children as psychotherapy patients.* American Psychological Association Meeting, New Orleans LA, 1974.

Stier, S. Children's rights and societies' duties, *Journal of Social Issues,* 1978, *34*(2), 46–58.

Tokanishi, R. Childhood as a social issue: Historical roots of contemporary child advocacy movements, *Journal of Social Issues,* 1978, *34*(2), 8–27.

United Nations, *Declaration of the Rights of the Child.* Adopted by the General Assembly, 1959.

The Tortious Evolution
of Patients' Rights

CHAPTER 4

BARBARA SMITH

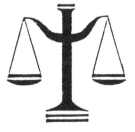

THE TORTIOUS EVOLUTION OF PATIENTS' RIGHTS

4

Barbara Smith

Within the context of the mental health professions, the rights of patients have been flagrantly abused as a result of involuntary commitment proceedings to mental hospitals. The American Psychiatric Association in March of 1961, submitted a statement of its position with respect to the "Constitutional Rights of the Mentally Ill" to the Senate Subcommittee on Constitutional Rights. In this statement, the APA asserted that, "We want to be considered doctors, not jailers. We know that. . .our patients react with the same rage as would any citizen, and such rage is not an auspicious starting point for treatment" (Szasz, 1973, p. 232).

However, as eloquently testified to by such writers as Szasz (1963; 1969), Ennis (1972) and Halleck (1969), traditional psychiatric hospitals have been nothing short of jails, where commitment has been equated with legal incompetence and a resulting deprivation of legal recourse to "habeas corpus."

Szasz pointed out, historically, why mentally ill patients have had such a battle in regaining rights guaranteed to all citizens by the constitution. The guarantees established by the constitution and its amendments apply only to persons involved in criminal proceedings, that is to say, individuals in conflict with the society at large or with the state (see ED. NOTE below.)

ED. NOTE: This statement by the author is not correct. The Due Process clauses of the Fifth and Fourteenth Amendments to the Constitution of the United States are applicable to individuals involved in civil commitment proceedings. See the decision of the U.S. Supreme Court in *O'Conner v. Donaldson,* 422 U.S. 563 (1975), cited by the author.)

Conflicts between individuals come within the realm of civil law and therefore supposedly do not require protection from governmental abuse of power. So long as courts have defined involuntary hospitalization and involuntary mental treatment as therapeutic and not punitive, legal proceedings have been considered civil rather than criminal. The person defined as patient has therefore lost the traditional constitutional guarantees which were established to protect the accused in criminal proceedings from possible governmental abuse of power. Indefinite commitment without judicial recourse as well as a policy of "guilty until proven innocent" without recourse to jury trial has therefore characterized civil commitment proceedings (see Szasz, 1963, Chapter 15).

In order to understand the rights of patients in the courts, it is imperative to understand the procedure of civil suits, the major form of suit brought against psychiatrists and psychotherapists. The most frequent form of civil suit is based on tort law, in which the plantiff seeks redress from another individual for sustained injuries of an economic, physical, or mental nature. The decisions in such civil suits are based on "common law," statutory law, or "case law," which is law created by prior cases. The judge must decide each case on the basis of whether or not it falls within the rule of common law, statute, prior case law, or whether new law should be declared based on the facts of the present case.

The Implications of *O'Connor v. Donaldson*

One of the most important precedent-setting cases for the rights of mental patients, with respect to involuntary hospitalization, was the 1975 case of *O'Connor v. Donaldson.* This decision by the U.S. Supreme Court arose in the State of Florida.

Kenneth Donaldson was committed in civil proceedings to confinement as a mental patient in the Florida State Hospital in January of 1957 and was kept in custody there for a period of nearly 15 years against his will, without treatment "designed to alleviate or cure his supposed illness," and despite undertakings by responsible persons to care for him.

The position of O'Connor, the superintendent of the hospital during Donaldson's confinement was his good faith reliance upon State Law, which he believed valid and which "had authorized indefinite custodial confinement of the 'sick' even if they were not treated and their release could harm no one." The case came before the U.S. Supreme Court on the appeal from a verdict in favor of Donaldson for $38,000 in damages assessed in a jury trial in the U.S. District Court. The principle findings by the Supreme Court subsequent to O'Connor's appeal were the following:

> The State may not confine the harmless mentally ill solely to save its citizens from exposure to those whose ways are different. . .Mere public intolerance or animosity cannot constitutionally justify the deprivation of a person's physical liberty (422 U.S. at p. 575).

> A State cannot constitutionally confine a nondangerous individual who is capable of surviving safely in freedom by himself or with the help of willing and responsible family members or friends (422 U.S. at p. 576).

This ruling touches on the issue of determining dangerousness as behavior distinct from differentness. In an intensive project directed at examination of the Administration of Psychiatric Justice in the state of Arizona, the Civil commitment Process was thoroughly questioned and summarized. In this review, concluding testimony from the subcommittee on Mental Health Service of the California State Legislature with respect to the prediction of dangerousness, pointed out that "with regard to potentially dangerous persons, the evidence available indicates that there are no tests that predict an individual's capacity for dangerous behavior" (Wexler, 1971, p. 97). Furthermore, Dershowitz reported from his survey of the literature on prediction of antisocial conduct that available studies "strongly suggest that psychiatrists are rather inaccurate predictors, inaccurate in an absolute sense, and even less accurate when compared with other professionals, such as psychologists, social workers, and correctional officials; and when compared to actuarial devices, such as prediction or experience tables (Derskowitz, 1969, p. 45).

In sum, psychiatrists are prone to follow the basic rule of "better safe than sorry," thereby overpredicting rather than underpredicting dangerousness, and consequently wrongfully depriving many individuals of their liberty. In another penetrating review of the literature on the reliability and validity of psychiatrist predictions of dangerousness, Ennis and Litwack (1974) presented studies that give estimates of false positives (the harmless predicted as dangerous) ranging from 65% to 95%.

The Supreme Court of the United States in a case, cited again by Bruce Ennis (*Minnesota ex rel. Pearson v. Probate Court*), suggested that "specific evidence of past misconduct is a constitutionally preferable test of future dangerousness, and may well be the only constitutionally adequate standard" (Referred to in Wexler, 1971, pp. 99–100). [See Ed. Note on following page].

The Arizona Project specifically singles out California's Lanterman-Petris-Short Act of 1969, California Welfare and Institutions Code, Sections 5150–5278) as representing a model for more stringent statutory standards. Here, in order for the patient to be held for the most extensive time period of 90 days, he must either have recently threatened, attempted or successfully inflicted physical harm upon another individual which resulted in his being taken into custody or have committed such acts while in custody and "as a result of mental disorder is an imminent threat of substantial physical harm to others" (California Welfare and Institutions Code, Section 5300).

The *O'Connor v. Donaldson* decision also discussed constitutional questions concerning the second traditional condition for confinement of the mentally ill; that is, the need for treatment, which is also questioned by Szasz (1963, p. 240) and Schwitzgebel (1974). However, the U.S. Supreme Court did not approve or use as a basis for its ruling the lower Court of Appeal holding that "a person involuntarily civilly committed to a mental hospital does have a constitutional right to receive such treatment as will give him a realistic opportunity to be cured" (see the concurring opinion of Chief Justice Burger at 422 U.S. 580).

As also discussed by Szasz, constitutionally, the right to treatment as a condition of commitment is seen as making up for the loss of the safeguards found in the criminal process, but not present in civil commitment. Chief Justice Burger's concurring

---

ED. NOTE: This interpretation of the U.S. Supreme Court's hold in *Minnesota ex rel. Pearson v. Probate Court* is not supported by a reading of the case. Pearson claimed Minnesota statutes providing commitment procedures for individuals suffering from "psychopathic personalities" deprived him of due process. The term "psychopathic personalities" was defined as including "those persons who, by an habitual course of misconduct in sexual matters, have evidenced an utter lack of power to control their sexual impulses and who, as a result, are likely to attack or otherwise inflict injury, loss, pain or other evil on the objects of their uncontrolled and uncontrollable desire." (309 U.S. at p. 273). The Court merely held that "evidence of past conduct pointing to probable consequences [is] as susceptible of proof as many of the criteria constantly applied in prosecutions for crime" (309 U.S. at p. 274). His appeal was rejected.

opinion in *O'Connor v. Donaldson*, vigorously disagrees with the lower Court of Appeal ruling quoted above, and points out that the justification of commitment, based on the right to treatment, is actually an intolerable interference with the right of the State as parens patriae to implement a particular scheme for protection of the mentally ill upon a legislative determination that it is in the best interest of the affected class and that its members are unable to act for themselves (422 U.S. at p. 583). The Chief Justice points out that many mentally ill persons are uncurable or reject treatment. Thus they cannot be given such treatment as will afford a realistic opportunity for cure (422, U.S. at p. 584).

Modes of Legal Recourse Within Hospitalized Settings

The majority of the cases brought to bear against psychiatrists within the hospital setting are on grounds of malpractice. For purposes of this discussion, the tort of malpractice may be summarized as a negligent deviation from the prevailing standard of care for the medical specialization of psychiatry. Damages recoverable may include losses for false imprisonment, and personal injuries, including mental and emotional anguish and suffering naturally flowing from the negligent act (see, for example the New York decision *Ferrara v. Gallucho*, ruling mental pain and anguish as actionable injury).

Some of the bases for claims against the therapist available to voluntary and involuntary hospitalized patients fall into the following categories:

(1) professional negligence as determined by lack of informed consent for treatment using mechanical or chemical therapeutic intervention;
(2) negligence with respect to restraining and controlling patients;
(3) negligence pertaining to the improper commitment of a person to a mental institution (false imprisonment).

Most frequently found with the first category, dealing with informed consent, are the electroshock cases. Physical injury has been a consequence to the treatment, and where the plaintiff-patient claims inadequate information as to the possible hazards, such that the patient could have made an informed decision as to whether to accept the risks of the treatment. *Woods v. Brumlop* is a court decision representative of such an action. The court concluded that "without full and frank disclosure to the patient by physician of all pertinent facts relative to his illness and treatment prescribed or recommended, any consent obtained from patient for administration of such treatment is ineffectual."

The second category deals with proper control and restraints, including appropriate controlling surveillance of suicide-prone patients. As established in the Colorado decision in *Bellandi v. Park Sanitarium Association*, the court held that "Institutions dealing with persons affected with nervous diseases should have reasonable devices of restraint and sufficient attendants to handle violent cases with minimum danger to the patient." Wrongful death due to a negligent and wrongful act was the judgment rendered against the Sanitarium and staff that used a towel tourniquet about the neck and large amounts of ether to restrain a patient who died in the midst of the "controlling procedures."

In *Kent v. Whitaker*, a state of Washington decision, negligence was established by the failure of the psychiatrist to use reasonable care in treating patients for their illness by failing to safeguard them from self-inflicted injury or death. This duty was held to be proper to the patient's needs and that such reasonable care and attention be furnished the patient as the patient's known mental condition requires (364 P.2d at p. 558). The patient in question, brought in because of a suicide attempt, was left alone in a locked room under the care of a nurse with 12 other patients to observe. Expert testimony was not considered necessary to establish that it was negligence on the part of the hospital staff which gave the patient the opportunity to kill herself.

Two other cases of the same nature are equally interesting in that the plaintiff lost, although a strong case for the plaintiff seemed apparent in each situation. In the Pennsylvania case of *Powell v. Risser*, even though the patient lost 60 percent usage of his hands as a result of wet-pack restraining procedures it was deemed through expert testimony, that treatment conformed to a "reasonable standard of care for that procedure." In *Dugan v. U.S.*, a District of Columbia case, the plaintiff died after being struck by another patient, whose pre-frontal lobotomy had defined him as "no longer assaultive." No clear and convincing evidence was found showing that the injury was caused by negligence or default of the institution or its agents. This decision points up the fact that negligence by the institution or the therapist must be found to exist before liability will exist. Injury alone is insufficient.

With respect to the third category, there are three main forms of recourse against improper commitment. The most difficult case to substantiate (10 percent success rate, p. 18, v. III, Hogan), focuses on the intention behind the diagnostic act in charges of malicious prosecution and libel or the malicious filing of a false affidavit asserting insanity. The second form of the third category of bases of law suits, and one somewhat more susceptible of substantiation, involves faulty psychiatric examination resulting in commitment. However Dawidoff describes the most effective legal weapon to be that of false imprisonment (20 percent success rate, p. 18, v. III, Hogan), which needs only proof of falseness rather than malice to be successful and when dealing with the police aspect of incarceration or deprivation of liberty, gives rise to arguments based on civil rights.

In concluding this cursory analysis of patient's rights with respect to hospitalization, it is noteworthy that, according to Hogan's survey of over 300 U.S. cases relevant to the practice of psychotherapy, plaintiffs have a better chance of receiving an award if the setting of the case is in a hospital, especially for verdicts of $25,000 or more (Hogan, v. III, p. 20).

The Rights of the Non-hospitalized Clients in Psychotherapy

While nearly two-thirds of all the 300 relevant U.S. Cases examined by Hogan occurred in hospital settings, and suits against private practitioners accounted for only 6.9 percent of all cases, there has been a gradual and consistent rise in malpractice actions filed as the public becomes more educated with respect to their rights and the psychotherapists' concomitant obligation to the patient.

Over 90 percent of all therapy cases involve torts of one sort or another, and, of those, over two-thirds concern the tort of malpractice. The cases of malpractice involving the therapist and client directly, bring into focus the primary legal nature of the therapeutic relationship as that of fiduciary and beneficiary. The sensitive duty of trust is crucial to the basic concept and process of therapy and defines the fiduciary responsibility of the therapist. Although, as in all tort law, the guidelines of conduct and actionable misconduct can only be established on a case-by-case basis, there are still primary guidelines to be followed. Dawidoff presents the fundamental guideline as that of requiring the fiduciary to prefer the interests of the beneficiary to his own.

Therapists can help ward off the possibility of malpractice litigation by maintaining a policy of continual honesty and self-scrutiny as to their own responses and motivations. Therapists have help in avoiding malpractice suits, not only through their own conscionable actions but also in the very nature of the procedure of malpractice litigation. It is difficult for the patient to establish a case of malpractice, as will become evident from the following brief analysis.

There are four essential elements to a malpractice action, all of which the patient must prove by a preponderance of the evidence. The plaintiff-patient must prove that: (1) a legal duty existed between the practitioner and the injured party; (2) that the practitioner was derelict in such duty; (3) that the patient subsequently suffered harm or injury of some sort, and: (4) that such harm was directly and proximately caused by the practitioner's dereliction or negligence of duty.

The first element normally presents no problem. However, the second element can be handled in one of two ways. Either expert testimony will be required or the principle of "res ipsa loquitur" (the thing speaks for itself) will apply. If an expert witness is necessary to determine dereliction of duty by a professional, the court will ask the following standard question:

> Did the practitioner conform to the standard of care required, measured by the degree of ability or skill possessed by other practitioners; the degree of care, attention, diligence, or vigilance ordinarily exercised by those practitioners in the application of their skills; and the special or extraordinary skill of specialists, if the practitioner has represented himself or herself, as such (U.S. DHEW, 1973a:123; see p.8, V.III, Hogan) (See ED. NOTE below)

ED. NOTE: Many states in applying the standard of care doctrine provide the therapist must only apply "that degree of learning and skill ordinarily possessed by reputable physicians and surgeons practicing in the same or a similar locality and under similar circumstances." See Calif. Jury Instruction, Civil (6th Ed.), p. 176, Instruction 6.00. cf. Instruction 6.37 id. p. 209 relative to the "Duty of a Professional" and Instructions 6.37.1 at id p. 211 on the "Duty of a Specialist." All use the phrase "in the same or similar locality and under similar circumstances."

As a result of this formulation of the standard of care, clinical psychologists will be judged only with respect to level of expertise of non-medical professionals in clinical psychology and the courts cannot require them to meet the standards of psychiatrists or physicians. However, one of the problems for the plaintiff within the overall field of psychotherapy is the determination of the particular school of therapy, and what are the appropriate standards of care of that school that the practitioner ought to adhere to, be they psychiatrist, psychologist, family therapist, etc. The courts have been and continue to be sensitive to the need for experimentation in the young and evolving profession of psychotherapy. Thus in newer treatment modalities, it is generally required that a respectable minority of the profession must adhere to such a line of thought (p. 9, v. III, Hogan).

Once the standard of care has been determined, it then becomes necessary to prove negligence within such a standard. Here, expert testimony is not required, although it certainly can help, and "the plaintiff may demonstrate negligence through written memoranda, letters and statements of witnesses" (p.10, v.III, Hogan). However, the client-plaintiff is at a distinct disadvantage with respect to acuity of perception in what are normally one-to-one contact sessions with the professional. The psychotherapist has not only the prestige of the profession as opposed to the label of patient, but various allegations by the patient of abuse (especially sexual), can always be attributed to neurotic or psychotic projective fantasies on the part of the patient. As summed up by Louisell and Williams:

> Proof or disproof of alleged details of a transaction between psychiatrist and a patient who actually requires psychiatric treatment perhaps constitutes one of the most difficult problems in medico-legal affairs (Louisell & Williams, 1977, p.51).

In such cases, the courts have to avoid the twin pitfalls of excessive sympathy for the patient as well as the over-estimation of the position of the psychotherapist.

While the client-plaintiff has recourse to the legal proceedings of malpractice, with respect to negligence on the part of the psychotherapist, this is not to say that every mistake in judgment is a cause for a malpractice action. In cases of merely erroneous professional judgment, "the courts will not generally grant a verdict for the plaintiff" (p.10, v.III, Hogan). Or, as Dawidoff expressed it, "negligence or breach of the duties of skill and care, may not be presumed from the fact of mistaken judgment" (Dawidoff, 1973, p. 71). (See ED. NOTE below)

In cases where negligence is so plain that a claim of non-negligence offends the basis common sense of the community, the procedure of expert testimony may well be dispensed with and the courts will apply the doctrine of *"res ipsa loquitur"* (For example, see the New York Court of Appeals in the case of *Hammer v. Rosen*).

One further problem, once deviation from standard of care on the part of the professional and actionable injury with respect to the client have been established, is proof the injury in question was "proximately" caused by the negligent activity. With all the welter of impinging life events contributing to the client's mental stability, in addition to the interaction with the professional, there is generally "extreme difficulty in proving proximate causation. . ." (p.11, v.III, Hogan). Here, expert testimony is once again relied upon, unless the negligence is so glaring as to be readily discernible to the average person as required for the application of the principal of *"res ipsa loquitur."* In general, "to sustain a cause of action for malpractice, there must be proof that improvement, of which there was substantial likelihood, was prevented by the psychiatrist's breach of duty" (Dawidoff, 1973, pp. 74–75).

Setting the Limits

Three court cases are generally cited as having successfully impacted the regulation of psychotherapeutic practices. The first and probably the most frequently mentioned is that of *Landau v.*

ED. NOTE: For example, in California, A physician, surgeon, psychotherapist, attorney or other professional or specialist is not negligent merely because his efforts prove unsuccessful or he errs in judgment. However, he is negligent if his lack of success or error in judgment is due to a failure to perform his duties. See California Jury Instructions, Civil (6th ed.) Instruction No. 6.02 (1981 Revision) and Instruction No. 6.37.2 (1981 Revision).

Werner (1961). (See. ED. NOTE below). In this case, the plaintiff, Landau, was a single, middle-aged, anxiety-ridden woman who developed deep feelings of love, obsession and bondage with her psychiatrist, Dr. Werner. Dr. Werner explained this as part of the process of "transference," and he advised plaintiff to continue treatment. After six months, it was decided to cease treatment, but, taking the view that a sudden withdrawal might cause a relapse, Dr. Werner decided on a series of innocent, friendly social contacts over some months, but he gradually withdrew from the relationship. Plaintiff relapsed, attempted suicide at the doctor's home. He resumed treatment in a final effort to resolve the transference, but terminated treatment when it had no effect. The judge determined that the doctor was not guilty of any misconduct. However, the judge found that the social contacts were admittedly a departure from standard practice in psychiatry. He pointed out that Dr. Werner "had explosive forces under his control and if a mistake were made, the consequences might be disasterous and irrevocable." The court found the departure from standard practice constituted negligence which resulted in gross deterioration in plaintiff's health and awarded plaintiff damages. Dr. Werner "acted almost disloyally by apparent attempt to reap personal satisfaction from the beneficiary of the fiduciary relationship" (Dawidoff, 1973, p.80).

Landau v. Werner provided the precedential legal opening for courts to potentially control any act which a psychotherapist employs in dealing with clients. While in this case, it was not a clear-cut question of a professional seeking purposeful personal satisfaction at the expense of the client, in another case arising in Missouri, *Zipkin v. Freeman* (1968), the psychiatrist, Freeman, was found to have been grossly negligent in his manipulative, exploitive behavior with respect to his patient, Mrs. Zipkin. Here again, the primary issue was the mishandling of the transference phenomenon, in which the patient professed love for the psychiatrist. Dr. Freeman not only did nothing to discourage Mrs. Zipkin's love for him personally, but entered into extensive social and financial relations with her in a clear attempt to render her

---

ED. NOTE: *Landau v. Werner* is a decision rendered in the Queen's Bench Division of the English Courts. The Queen's Bench Division is the English equivalent of the American trial court of general jurisdiction.

even more dependent upon him as a necessary condition of her successful "therapy."

While Freeman was charged with malpractice based on negligent and improper therapy, a question was raised on appeal as to whether the acts of socializing could really be considered part of professional services. Freeman's insurance company initially refused to pay damages levied against him on the grounds that his activities and conduct went outside of the framework of professional services, thereby excluding them from the terms of coverage of the policy. The court ruled, however, that based on expert testimony, those actions taken by Freeman fundamentally violated standards of care for proper therapy, rather than being irrelevant to therapy. As in the previous case, the court directed that psychotherapists "should not enter into social relations with the patient if he wants her to improve; that the transference phenomenon is why treatment should be handled in the office. . ." (*Zipkin v. Freeman*, 436 S.W. 2d at p. 760).

In the third case, *Hammer v. Rosen*, the New York court addressed itself, not to behavior that went beyond the bounds of therapy, but a specific mode of therapy itself. The plaintiff, Alice Hammer, was a patient with schizophrenia, treated for seven years by Dr. Rosen, a psychiatrist. The plaintiff brought three witnesses to establish that she had been beaten on a number of different occasions by Dr. Rosen, as part of her therapy. No expert testimony was required to establish evidence of malpractice, because "the very nature of the acts complained of bespeaks improper treatment and malpractice" (*Hammer v. Rosen,* 165 S.E. 2d 756 at p. 757).

Unfortunately, Dr. Rosen, apparently as a trial tactic, chose not to defend his actions on the grounds of defendable therapy practice, even though he had published work on a theory of physical confrontation as a means of treating schizophrenia. Instead, during the trial, he abandoned all clinical defense of his therapy, even acknowledging in a court brief, "that any mode of treatment which involves assaults upon the patient is 'fantastic' ". Therefore, the court never had to deal with the issue of establishing a standard of care for an innovative therapeutic practice and what its position would have been on such grounds was left essentially unclear. However, the court still took a definite stand on establishing limits to experiment with therapeutic modalities. In essence, the court declared through the principle of "*res ipsa loquitur*," that no physical beating of patients could be considered a legitimate therapeutic task. As Dawidoff pointed out, "the judicial message may have been that psychotherapy was at last subjected to being governed in malpractice" (Dawidoff, 1973, p. 79).

These three cases demonstrate that courts are willing to place legal restraints on the practice of psychotherapy and establish definite boundaries beyond which the psychotherapist cannot go with a client.

In addition to the courtroom litigation concerning therapeutic practice, the courts have also examined the duties and rights of the fiduciary-beneficiary relationship with respect to the critical area of confidentiality. Three major cases highlight the position of courts on a concept which is integral to the basic endeavor of psychotherapy.

The California legislature has enacted into law the duty of the psychotherapist not to disclose matters related to him/her in confidence (Evidence Code, Section 1012). Evidence Code, Section 1014 provides, in part, that "the patient, whether or not a party, has a privilege to refuse to disclose, and prevent another from disclosing, a confidential communication between patient and psychotherapist." However, Evidence Code, Section 1024 creates a specific and limited exception to such privilege stating that there is no privilege "if the psychotherapist has reasonable cause to believe that the patient is in such mental or emotional condition as to be dangerous to himself or to the person or property of another and that disclosure of the communication is necessary to prevent the threatened danger." In a more succinct rendering of the exception, it may be said that "protective privilege ends where the public peril begins" (*Tarasoff v. Regents*, 17 Cal. 2d 425 at p. 442).

As illuminated by Fleming and Maximov, *Tarasoff v. Regents* essentially tested the implications of Evidence Code Section 1024 as to whether it established merely right to disclose or duty to disclose. The case revolved around the murder of Tatiana Tarasoff by a former patient of a psychotherapist employed by the University of California. While the patient had been briefly detained by campus police after threatening the life of Tatiana, neither the parents, nor the girl herself had ever been given warning by the psychotherapist. The court ruled that:

> A doctor or a psychotherapist treating a mentally ill patient, just as a doctor treating physical illness, bears a duty to use

reasonable care to give threatened persons such warnings
as are essential to avert foreseeable danger arising from his
patient's condition or treatment, when the psychotherapist
has reasonable cause to believe that the patient is in such a
mental or emotional condition as to be dangerous to himself
or to the person and property of another and that disclosure
of the communication is necessary to prevent the threatened
danger (see the Court's discussion, commencing at 17
Cal.3d, at p. 439).

The ruling emanating from the above case has not passed
without critical comment. Justice Clark, in his strong, well-
reasoned dissenting opinion, made several crucial points (made
elsewhere by A.A. Stone, 1976, and Fleming and Maximov, 1974).
Basically his opinion was that in imposing such duties on psychiatrists, the majority ruling actually contributes to society's
danger. With the difficulty, agreed to by all, in accurately predicting violence, the psychotherapist will both overpredict to avoid
his/her own civil peril and will avoid taking potentially violent
clients. With respect to the client, potentially violent people will
be deterred from seeking help or deterred from total self-
revelation, once in therapy, thereby crippling the underlying rapport of confidence and trust necessary for effective treatment
(see A.A. Stone, 1976, 17 Cal.3d at p. 452). As one safeguard to
both therapist and client, Fleming and Maximov stress the role
that "informed consent" can play at the beginning of therapy in
explaining the limits of confidentiality and the implicit risk of
disclosures beyond agreed limits.

A further exception to the requirement of confidentiality and
invalidating the notion of absolute privilege of confidentiality between client and psychotherapist is the rule in the California case
In Re Lifschutz. In this case, the psychotherapist, Lifschutz, was
held in custody for contempt of court after refusing on grounds
of absolute privilege to disclose confidential information relating
to a former patient. The particular circumstances of the case that
convinced the court to assert that "no constitutional right
enables psychotherapists to assert absolute privilege concerning
all psychotherapy communications," (p. 830), was the fact that
the patient had initiated the litigation during which he voluntarily
disclosed his former relationship with the psychotherapist and
this information regarding his emotional-mental condition
became critical to his pleadings. Therefore, the court ruled that

when the patient voluntarily gives information relating to the patient-psychotherapist relationship in litigation he has initiated, then the therapist is compelled to make exception and disclose those confidential matters thus referred to by the patient. The principle is that once the confidence has been disclosed there is no longer a confidence to protect.

Lastly, the Utah case of *Berry v. Moench* (1958, 33 P.2d 814), qualifies the extent of the disclosure and points out the libelous pitfalls of too indiscreet a disclosure. Patient-plaintiff, Berry, brought action against Dr. Moench for having disclosed information about his treatment in a letter secured by the physician of his fiancée's parents with respect to his mental-emotional health. As a result of the information in the letter, the girl's parents disinherited her after she insisted on pursuing her marriage plans with the patient despite their strenuous objections. The court ruled that conditional privilege did exist in the interest of protecting a third party, but only under the following conditions. Disclosure must be "exercised in good faith, resonable care must be exercised as to its truth, information must be fairly reported, and only such information should be conveyed and only to such persons as is necessary to the purpose" (331 P2d at p. 215). Should these conditions be violated, grounds for charges of libel could be present.

Impact of Litigation on Patient-Client Rights

Overall, the total number of suits against therapists is small, although the figure is steadily rising. Difficulty of establishing proof of malpractice as well as the mean length of time of 4.8 years from negligent act to final decision (Hogan, 1979, v.III, p.22), tend to reduce the frequency of cases. In addition, there are the natural built-in safeguards of the therapeutic procedure which include expectation and appropriate skills for handling hostility and other negative feelings. And finally as pointed out by Hogan, among others, patients who have been harmed are often loath to disclose the details surrounding the incident in a court of law (Hogan, 1979, v.I, p.320).

With regard to the overall impact of malpractice suits in psychotherapy, while beneficial legal effects have certainly occurred in the realm of patient rights in the hospital setting, with respect to the client vis-a-vis the private practitioner, the impact on client rights is more controversial.

The possible negative outcomes for psychotherapy as a result of the Tarasoff ruling have already been mentioned. Two further points have been made with respect to the overall effect of malpractice suits on the quality of professional practice.

With the exceptions of the types of cases already mentioned, so long as therapists confine themselves to verbal interventions, "they will remain relatively immune from suit, no matter how poor their advice, how damaging their comments, or how incorrect their interpretations" (Hogan, v.I, p.322). Furthermore, litigation remains hopelessly ineffectual for controlling those therapists who are the most irresponsible and dangerous, because it is typically those less qualified and uncredentialed therapists who are not worth suing since they are not covered by insurance.

Finally, judicial regulation of psychotherapy is fraught with difficulty and "the courts must tread carefully in attempting to establish standards of practice" in a young field subject to continual innovation and experimentation (Hogan, v.I, p. 323). At least, the courts have taken a decided stand in favor of assuring civil liberties to those labeled "mentally ill" in hospital settings and although the effects on the therapeutic relationship are still to be assessed, the courts have also assured the client-plaintiff that psychotherapists are subject to legal restraints in their practice and confidential disclosures.

REFERENCES

Dawidoff, D. *The Malpractice of Psychiatrists*, Springfield IL: C.C. Thomas, 1973.

Derskowitz, A. The psychiatrist's power in civil commitment: A knife that cuts both ways, *Psychology Today*, February 1969, 2(9), 43–47.

Ennis, B. *Prisoners of Psychiatry*, NY: Avon Books, 1972.

Ennis, B. & Litwack, T. Psychiatry and the presumption of expertise: Flipping coins in the courtroom, *62 Calif. Law Rev.*, 1974, 693.

Fleming, J. & Maximov, B. The patient or his victim: The therapist dilemma, *62 Calif. Law Rev.*, 1974, 1025.

Halleck, S. The psychiatrist and the legal process, *Psychology Today*, February 1969, 2(9), 25–28.

Halleck, S. The reform of mental hospitals, *Psychology Today*, March 1969, 2(10, 50–51.

Hogan, D. *The Regulation of Psychotherapist: A study of the Philosophy and Practice of Professional Regulation, Vol. 1,* 315–327; and *A Review of Malpractice Suits in the U.S., Vol.III,* 7–27. Cambridge Mass: Ballinger Publishing Co., 1979.

Louisell, D. & Williams, H. *Trial of Medical Malpractice Cases,* NY: Matthew Bender, 1977, Paragraph 2.16.

Schwitzgebel, R. The right to effective mental treatment, *62 Calif. Law Rev.,* 1974, 936.

Morse, H. The tort liability of the psychiatrist, *Syracuse Law Review,* Summer 1967, *18*(4), 691–727.

Stone, A. The Tarasoff decision: Suing psychotherapists to safeguard society, *90 Harvard Law Review,* 1976, 358).

Szasz, T. *Law, Liberty and Psychiatry,* NY: Collier Books, 1963.

Szasz, T. (Ed.) Position statement on the medical treatment of the mentally ill, *The Age of Madness.* NY: Anchor Books, 1973.

Szasz, T. The crime of commitment, *Psychology Today,* March 1969, 2(10), 55–57.

Wexler, D. & Scovill, S. Administration of psychiatric justice, *Arizona Law Review,* 1971, *13*, 4–15, 77–83, 97–113.

CASES CITED

Bellandi v. Park Sanitarium Ass'n, 214 Cal. 488, 6 P.2d 508 (1931).

Berry v. Moench, 8 U.2d 191, 331 P.2d 814 (1958).

Dugan v. U.S., District of Columbia, 147 F. Supp. 674 (1956).

Ferrara v. Gallucho, 5 N.Y.2d 16 (Ct. Opp.), 165 N.E.2d 249 (1958).

Hammer v. Rosen, 7 N.Y.2d 376, 165 N.E.2d 756 (1960).

In Re Lifschutz, 2 C.3d 415, 467 P.2d 557 (1970).

Kent v. Whitaker, 58 Wash.2d 569, 364 P.2d 556 (1961).

Landau v. Werner, 105 Solicitor's Journal 1008 (1961).

O'Connor v. Donaldson, 422 U.S. 563, 45 L.Ed.2d 596, 95 S.Ct. 2486 (1975).

Minnesota ex rel. Pearson v. Probate Court of Ramsey County, 309 U.S. 270 (1940).

Powell v. Risser, 375 Pa. 60, pp A.2d 454 (1953).

Tarasoff v. The Regents of the University of California, 529 P.2d 553 (1974); 17 C.3d 425 (1976).

Woods v. Brumlop, 71 N.M. 221, 377 P.2d 520 (1962).

Zipkin v. Freeman, 436 S.W.2d 753 (1968).

Children of Divorce:
The Interweaving of Legal and Psychological Issues

CHAPTER 5

VICKI NEVINS

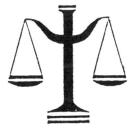

CHILDREN OF DIVORCE: THE INTERWEAVING OF LEGAL AND PSYCHOLOGICAL ISSUES

5

Vicki Nevins

> Children of divorce are among the most abused members of society. They are the quiet victims of a devastating process which inevitably creates sheer havoc in their lives. . . . Our legal system has unfortunately perpetuated the myth that the parties to a divorce action include only the husband, wife, and the court (Anderson, 1977, p.41).

Divorce is a serious crisis for all involved parties and it can have tremendous repercussions on a child's emotional development. Although such disruption may be ameliorated by appropriate legal and psychological interventions, the legal and mental health professions often neglect the needs of the child of divorce.

Despite the principle of "best interests of the child," the legal profession has been criticized for inflicting psychological damage on children due to the nature of the adversary process. Similarly, the mental health profession has sometimes been guilty of serving the needs of attorneys and parents, while giving little attention to the children of divorce.

Fortunately, our knowledge about the effectiveness of the various alternatives to the adversary process is expanding, as is our knowledge of the special needs of the child of divorce. The concept of fault has recently been cited as being both ineffective and destructive to the child's best interests. Recent legislation in California and the concept of mediation counseling as a viable alternative to litigation may well aid families and the legal system to resolve the conflicts engendered by divorce in an effective and constructive manner.

Legal and psychological issues are interwoven in the fabric of the divorce process (Henning & Oldham, 1977). Experts in the field have pointed out the difference between "legal divorce" and "emotional divorce" (Despert, 1953; Elkin, 1977). The number of cases of disputed custody is rising. Custody and visitation disputes are expensive and continue for years. Frequently, they are detrimental to the mental health of children (Taylor & Werner, 1978). Postdivorce litigation regarding custody and visitation is often a smokescreen for the real problem, which is that the spouses are still very much connected by anger and other emotions.

Often the legal process is used as an instrument by one parent to harass the other, and the child becomes a pawn in the long bargaining process of divorce. The normal fears of the child of divorce (abandonment fears, guilt, responsibility) are exacerbated by the legal issues. Some critics of the legal system have gone so far as to state that the typical negative reactions of children of divorce represent merely an adjustment to circumstances where their best interests have been ignored (Salk, 1977). The major problem seems to be the lack of consensus among the experts as to what really is in the best interests of the child.

Fortunately, the American legal approach regarding child custody determinations is currently undergoing a significant change, especially in states such as California. Under English common law, custody of a child was considered a property right. Custody was automatically granted to the father, with no consideration given to the best interest of the child. Judicial attitudes toward custody gradually changed with changing social trends and the rule evolved that mothers got custody of daughters while fathers were awarded custody of sons, unless the boys were very young.

California recognized the "tender years doctrine" for many years. Under former Civil Code Section 138, which was in effect until 1970, young children were given to the mother, while the father was given custody of a child of an age to require education and preparation for labor/business. In practice, though, the father's claim to custody was generally upheld (Roeder, 1979). In 1970, California adopted a new Family Law Act to create "no-fault divorce."

Section 4600 of the Civil Code was modified to state that custody be awarded to *either* parent according to the "best interests of the child," but, other things being equal, to the mother if the child was of "tender years." Section 4600 was amended in 1972, to delete the preference for mothers of young children over fathers, in custody litigation. Nevertheless, many fathers' rights advocates claimed that mothers continued to be awarded custody more than 90 percent of the time (Roman & Haddad, 1978).

Some 85 militant fathers' rights groups around the country have recently become an influential force determined to bring about changes in child custody laws (Ware, 1980). Such advocates of fathers' rights complain that the mother's courtroom advantage violates the 14th Amendment's guarantee against sexual discrimination (Roman & Haddad, 1978). Others have complained that the law gave too much latitude and discretion to judges who frequently held archaic attitudes about family matters (Salk, 1977; Silver, 1978). These critics of the legal system have argued that social customs, unsupported by scientific facts, led judges to favor mothers, a practice which deprives children and fathers of their constitutional right to due process of law while promoting negative psychological consequences. It could also be argued that the lack of consideration given to the preference of children under the age of 14 violates their constitutional rights.

In January of 1980, Section 4600 was again modified to state that custody be awarded to *both* parents jointly or to either parent, while specifically stating that custody awards should not be based on the parent's sex. This new law begins by stating:

> . . . the legislature finds and declares that it is the public policy of this state to assure minor children of frequent and continuous contact with both parents after the parents have separated or dissolved their marriage, and to encourage parents to share the rights and responsibilities of child rearing in order to effect this policy.

In addition, Section 4600.5 has been added to the Civil Code, stating that "joint custody is in the best interests of a minor child" when the parents so agree. If either parent requests joint custody, the court must now grant it or else state the reasons for denial. This is a significant change in policy and seems to have had a significant impact on the number of joint custody awards in California (Beasley, 1980). More than a dozen other states now have similar joint custody statutes (Folberg, 1980). Nevertheless, there is still much controversy surrounding the new law and a lack of consensus among experts as to whether or not joint custody is in the best interests of the child.

The controversy regarding the ability of the legal profession to determine the child's best interests is well illustrated by the publication of *Beyond the Best Interest of the Child* (Goldstein, Freud, & Solnit, 1973). These well-respected authors protested the "reasonable visitation" clause that is written into divorce statutes in most states, and thereby had a considerable influence on family law. This book strongly recommended that one parent have total management and control of custody, since "continuity" was cited to be a crucial need of the child. Since visitation was viewed as a potential source of discontinuity, these authors stated that the "non-custodial parent should have no legally enforceable right to visit the child" (Goldstein, Freud, & Solnit, 1973, p.38).

This recommendation, which seems to be based on no scientific evidence, infuriated many non-custodial fathers. Recent research has argued against this notorious book by establishing that frequent access to the non-custodial parent is favored by children of divorce and is a significant factor in promoting their psychological health (Rosen, 1977; Wallerstein & Kelly, 1980). Wallerstein and Kelly's (1980) important study found that the three major characteristics of children who coped best with divorce were free access to the non-custodial parent, diminished hostility between the former spouses, and the child's realistic understanding of the divorce. It seems crucial to the child's psychological well-being that he or she understand that the parents are divorcing each other, not the child. It appears that it is the responsibility of both the legal and mental health professions to put this new knowledge into practice.

Joint custody is a new and controversial concept, lauded by some and denigrated by others. Although personal accounts of joint physical custody (Galper, 1978; Ware, 1980; my own personal experience) and one research study (Abarbanel, 1977) support the psychological benefits on children of such arrangements. One recent study (Steinman, 1980), as yet unpublished, found ambivalent results (i.e., joint custody was good for most children but anxiety-provoking for others).

In any case, there seems to be little evidence to support the view of Goldstein, Freud, and Solnit (1973) that visitation could be psychologically detrimental due to the child's need for continuity. The major problem with joint custody, as espoused by its many critics, is that it simply is unworkable in most cases due to the inability of the former spouses to cooperate in the joint venture of childrearing (Fainer & Wasser, 1980; Roeder, 1979). Such authors have questioned how joint custody can be in the child's best interest since it divides authority between former spouses who are at war with each other, making it more likely that the child will be used as a weapon.

Rather than having the legal profession force joint custody arrangements, it seems to be more advisable to have the mental health profession help parents to accept emotionally the importance of the child's access to both parents. Conciliation courts in California and several other states are dedicated to the principle of aiding parents, through counseling, to put aside their own hostility for the sake of the child and work out custodial arrangements which truly reflect the child's best interests (Elkin, 1979; Taylor & Werner, 1978).

Unfortunately, as of 1977, only 15 of 58 counties in California had such conciliation courts. Nevertheless, new legislation in California (Senate Bill 961, effective January, 1981) mandated mediation counseling in all cases of disputed custody and visitation. This new law seems to be an important step toward meeting the needs of the child of divorce.

Joint custody legislation is not a panacea for the problems of children of divorce. Legislation cannot mandate parents to stop using their children as weapons on the battleground of divorce. Legislation cannot force bitter and resentful parents to become friends in order to make the divorce easier for the children. Legislation cannot dispel the underlying dynamics of post-divorce conflicts, and it is these underlying issues, rather than the legal divorce per se, which are so damaging to the child.

With the impact of "no-fault divorce," parties can now vent their anger and hostility in court primarily in the arena of custody and visitation conflicts (Elkin, 1979). Visitation and custody conflicts are one way that divorced couples remain intensely attached (Chase, 1979; Tessman, 1978). Battles about the children are often "battles of involvement" and efforts to hold onto the past. Litigation is a long and costly process which cannot help but be psychologically damaging for the child, who feels the need to "take sides" in the fight. The continued conflict of the parents reinforces the child's anger, feelings of helplessness, guilt, and abandonment fears, while it also reinforces fantasies of reconciliation. The concept of "winners" and "losers" in custody battles cannot help but have serious negative effects on a child's self-esteem. "When a child is chronically exposed to the need of one parent to bolster the self by damaging the other parent . . . his ability to value himself in relation to identification figures cannot help but suffer" (Tessman, 1978, p. 321).

In addition to being an outlet for hostility, custody battles may also reflect the dependence of the adult on the child and the adult's need to hold on to the child to maintain his or her psychological balance (Wallerstein & Kelly, 1980). Children are often overwhelmed by the sense of power that such conflicts give them. Children are also frequently overwhelmed by the awesome sense of power and responsibility given to them when they are questioned regarding their custody preference. The anxiety which is evoked from having to decide between two significant figures can be psychologically traumatizing (Chase, 1980).

The legal profession rarely consults young children regarding their custody preference. When older children are consulted (usually in the judge's chambers), their preference is usually given little weight. Ferguson (1975) has argued that judges are often unskilled in the counseling techniques necessary to determine a child's true feelings. For this same reason, Chase (1980) has recommended using mental health consultants to interview children, believing that mental health professionals may be less likely than judges to ask parental preference questions which are undermining and anxiety-provoking.

Like custody battles, the underlying dynamics of visitation disputes make litigation unsuccessful. Children may develop a "visitation phobia" due to a fear of taking sides or an acting out of the custodial parent's anger (Chase, 1979). Such children cannot be forced by the court to visit their non-custodial parent. Similarly, custodial parents who deny visitation as a weapon to harass their former spouse may not be receptive to court orders. Many professionals in the field have recommended that "reasonable visitation" rights be set forth in more detail when there is much hostility between the parents (Henning & Oldham, 1977; Rosen, 1977). This standard phrase, "reasonable visitation," in divorce decrees is often abused due to insufficient clarity and definition.

Conciliation courts provide an important service in helping non-communicating couples specify exact visitation hours. The recommendation for flexibility in visitation plans is not that simple to provide, however, in the typical 3-hour intervention in a conciliation court. In addition, it is noteworthy that conciliation courts do not typically include the children in visitation conferences nor do they provide any interventions directed specifically at children. Preliminary results of a study recently completed at San Diego County's Conciliation Court (Nevins, 1981) indicated the need for such interventions with children.

The importance of seeking alternatives to litigation in resolving custody and visitation disputes cannot be overemphasized. The sooner such disputes end, the better (Elkin, 1979). The legal profession, by utilizing the adversary process, actually prolongs the conflict at the expense of the child's psychological well-being. Although lawyers may profess the child's interest, in practice they support their client's position, even if it is not in the best interest of the child (Gardner, 1977). Gardner (1977) has stated that custody battles in which lawyers enlist the aid of mental health professionals to prove their point rather than to learn what is best for the child are a disgrace to both professions. He has also argued that mental health professionals should warn their clients to avoid litigation in custody disputes and impress them with the right of self-determination.

Finally, Gardner states that lawyers must be viewed as servants and advisors rather than individuals who rule parents in making custody decisions. Elkin (1977) argued that since children learn coping skills from parents, the courts have a responsibility to help divorced couples cope by providing counseling and educational services. California's conciliation courts have a success rate of 50 percent in helping parents work out self-determined custody and visitation agreements (Elkin, 1977).

Although it is apparent that the legal and mental health professions must cooperate in determining the best interests of the child in the divorce process, Swerdlow (1978) found that more than 50 percent of attorneys and judges do not use mental health services. This is alarming since the legal profession may not be sufficiently skilled in determining the child's best interest psychologically. Attorneys rarely ask what the child thinks of various proposed arrangements. When parents ask for legal advice in interpreting "reasonable visitation" rights, they are generally told that twice a month is standard (Wallerstein & Kelly, 1980). Sensitivity to the special needs and feelings of the child of divorce can only come about by increased cooperation of the legal and mental health professions. Senate Bill 961, which became effective in California in January of 1981, provided mandatory counseling in all cases of disputed custody and visitation. This legislation was an important step in mitigating the negative effects of such disputes on the psychological well-being of children.

The literature is replete with recommendations to ease the problems of the child of divorce. Most of the recommendations give priority to increased cooperation between the legal and mental health professions. Taylor and Werner (1978) recommended that there be conciliation courts in every county and training in the behavioral sciences for judges and attorneys. Some have recommended the appointment of counsel for children (Mnookin, 1978) or the use of a child advocate in all divorce proceedings (Anderson, 1977).

Henning and Oldham (1977) recommended psychological interventions to assure children of divorce that they are not being abandoned, are not to blame, etc. Fredericks (1976) argued for a new role for mental health professionals involved in custody battles: "explorer" instead of traditionalist. Unlike the traditionalist, whose function ends with the end of the marriage, the explorer counsels parents to help them separate emotionally and often works directly with the children, attempting to determine the relationship between the child and the custody seekers. Elkin (1977) suggested getting rid of words such as custody, visitation, and non-custodial, which keep us connected to outdated traditions. The granting of visitation rights to grandparents has also been suggested (Henning & Oldham, 1977; Gardner, 1977).

Most experts in the field of divorce have stressed the importance of post-divorce counseling in mitigating the hostility and tension of the spouses in order to promote the psychological growth of the children. Therapeutic interventions directed specifically at the children of divorce, although recommended by some, does not seem to be generally regarded as a top priority.

REFERENCES

Abarbanel, A. *Joint custody families: A case study approach.* Doctoral dissertation. San Diego: California School of Professional Psychology, 1977.

Anderson, H. Children of divorce, *Journal of Clinical Child Psychology, 6,* Summer 1977, 41–44.

Beasley, W. *Joint custody: 10 months down the line.* Los Angeles: 4th Annual Family Law Colloquium, November 1980.

Chase, G. *Visitation phobia.* Los Angeles: 2nd Annual Colloquium on Child Custody and Visitation, 1979.

Chase, G. *Criteria for psychiatric evaluations in child custody contests.* Los Angeles: 4th Annual Family Law Colloquium, 1980.

Despert, J. *Children of divorce.* Garden City NY: Dolphin Books, 1953.

Elkin, M. Postdivorce counseling in a conciliation court, *Journal of Divorce, 1,* Fall 1977, 55-65.

Elkin, M. *Custody and visitation: A time for change.* Los Angeles: 2nd Annual Colloquium on Child Custody and Visitation, 1979.

Fainer, R. & Wasser, D. *Child custody and visitation disputes: An overview.* Los Angeles: 4th Annual Family Law Colloquium, 1980.

Ferguson, P. Kids caught in custody, *Conciliation Court Review, 13,* 1975, 10-11.

Folberg, J. *The changing family: Implications for the law.* Los Angeles: 4th Annual Family Law Colloquium, 1980.

Fredericks, M. Custody battles: Mental-health professionals in the courtroom. In G. Koocher (Ed.), *Children's Rights and the Mental Health Professions.* NY: John Wiley & Sons, 1976.

Galper, M. *Co-parenting: Sharing your child equally.* Philadelphia: Running Press, 1978.

Gardner, R. Children of divorce: Some legal and Psychological considerations, *Journal of Clinical Child Psychology, 6,* 1977, 3-6.

Goldstein, J., Freud, A., & Solnit, A. *Beyond the best interest of the child.* NY: Free Press, 1973.

Henning, J. & Oldham, J. Children of divorce: legal and psychological crises. *Journal of Clinical Child Psychology, 6,* Summer 1977, 55-59.

Mnookin, R. & Kornhauser, L. Bargaining in the shadow of the law: The case of divorce, *The Yale Law Journal, 88,* 1979, 950.

Nevins, V. *The evaluation of the effectiveness of a group-treatment intervention with children of divorce.* Doctoral dissertation. San Diego: United States International University, 1981.

Roeder, E. *Joint custody: What is it? Where is it going? Will it work?* Los Angeles: 2nd Annual Colloquium on Child Custody and Visitation, 1979.

Roman, M. & Haddad, W. *The disposable parent: The case for joint custody.* NY: Holt, Rinehart, & Winston, 1978.

Rosen, R. Children of divorce: What they feel about access and other aspects of the divorce experience, *Journal of Clinical Child Psychology, 6,* Summer 1977, 24-27.

Salk, L. On the custody rights of fathers in divorce, *Journal of Clinical Child Psychology, 6,* Summer 1977, 49–51.

Steinman, S. *The Joint Custody Research Project.* Los Angeles: 4th Annual Family Law Colloquium, 1980.

Swerdlow, E. Mental health services available to the bench and bar to assist resolving problems relating to custody and visitation in family law cases, *Journal of Clinical Child Psychology, 7,* Fall 1978, 174–177.

Taylor, L. & Werner, E. Child custody and the conciliation courts, *Conciliation Courts Review, 16,* September 1978, 76–83.

Tessman, L. *Children of parting parents.* NY: Jason Aronson, 1978.

Wallerstein, J. & Kelly, J. *Surviving the break-up: How parents and children cope with divorce.* NY: Basic Books, 1980.

Ware, C. *Joint custody: One way to end the war.* Los Angeles: 4th Annual Family Law Colloquium, 1980.

ED.NOTE: California Senate Bill 961 cited in the text is found in the California Civil Code, Section 4607.

The Lesbian Mother:
A Struggle for Child Custody

CHAPTER 6

ANN BONNER

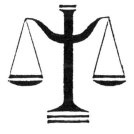

THE LESBIAN MOTHER: A STRUGGLE FOR CHILD CUSTODY

6

Ann Bonner

The purpose of this chapter is to provide an understanding of child custody laws in general, and their specific application to the lesbian mother who chooses to enter into a custody dispute for her child. An attempt will be made to elucidate the various concepts, laws, and applicable cases relating to custody and the lesbian mother and to postulate the possible impact on and implications for the lesbian mother, who attempts to obtain custody of her child.

"One-fifth of all lesbians and one-tenth of all gay men have children and the vast majority perform quite adequately as parents" (Riddle, 1978, p.44). One out of every ten women is a lesbian, according to Kingdon (1979). The most destructive and hurtful discrimination against gay people takes place in the realm of child custody. Many homosexuals are not only denied custody, but unfair visitation procedures are levied against them under the guise of being in the "best interests of the child." Publicized custody victories for gay parents give society the false impression that it is becoming a trend, which is definitely not the case. It is not uncommon for a lesbian mother to "win" a custody case with the stipulation that she is prohibited from living with her lover (Vida, 1978).

The Lesbian Mothers' National Defense Fund has been referred approximately 200 lesbian mother custody cases to date. Of these, one-third were settled out of court and custody was awarded to the mothers (Gibson, 1977). Some mothers chose not to fight; some of them did not have to. In the following pages we will examine some of the legal and ethical implications lesbian mothers face and the impact of these upon her.

An Evolving Concept: The Fitness Test

Two concepts that were traditionally applied in order to make a determination in child custody cases were the "fitness test" and the "tender years" concept. Based on a psychosocial approach to personality, a parent labeled "unfit" could be denied custody. The concept was open-ended and vague, but an unfit parent, usually meaning an unfit mother, came under one of five categories: nymphomaniac, alcoholic, child abuser, mentally ill, or a lesbian (McFadden, 1974).

In 1970, in California, with the passing of the Family Law Act, the parental preference doctrine or "fitness" concept was dropped and "finding of parental unfitness is no longer required by law . . . but it is closely related to the question of the best interest of the child . . . (Mills, 1979). However, a "statutory presumption of parent's unfitness is unconstitutional" (Mills, 1979, citing *Stanley v. Illinois*, 405 U.S. 645, 1972).

Twelve states, including California, concur with the Massachusetts Court's statement that the concept of the child's best interests and parental fitness are "cognate and connected" (Smith, 1979). In contrast, Woody (1978) stated that no attempt is made today to establish fitness or unfitness and that most states are now relying on a "better fit" conception.

Implications for the Lesbian Mother

Although California law has declared that the concept of fitness per se is unconstitutional, it still seems to be incorporated in or implicitly understood to be part of the presently supported "best interest of the child" doctrine.

In a 1974 California Supreme Court decision, In re B.G. (Mnookin, 1975) the term "unfit" was still applied in the California Court's statement in which a natural parent although judged to be not "unfit" could still be deprived of custody with custody awarded to a nonparent, if award of custody to a parent would be harmful to the child.

The Doctrine of Tender Years

The Talfourd Act of 1839, in espousing the concept of "parens patriae," set the stage for the formation of the "tender years" doctrine. Under the idea of parens patriae, the court was authorized as a "wise parent" to render a custody decision for a child under seven years of age (Franklin, 1980). In *Hart v. Hart* (Franklin, 1980), the tender years presumption was first set forth by the courts in 1880 and has managed to survive even today in some legal decisions (*Anderson v. Anderson*; Alexander, 1977). The Florida Statute 61.13 (2) provides that equal consideration be given to the father in custody cases. However, in *Anderson v. Anderson,* a Florida court in 1975 awarded a mother custody, stating that, if an infant is of "tender years," the mother should receive primary consideration.

In 1977, Pennsylvania publicly abolished the "tender years" concept (*Schall v. Schall*). Under the 1970 Family Law Act, the California Court stated that a woman should be given preference of "tender years" (Vida, 1978). In 1972, California abolished the mother's preference as to very young children.

Michigan courts seem to parallel California in abolishing the tender years concept. Until 1971, it was required that a child under twelve years of age be awarded to the mother (Benedek, 1979). In 1970, the Child Custody Act dropped the "tender years" concept and espoused the "best interest of the child" doctrine, listing ten factors to be taken into account including the preference of the child.

However, the "tender years" concept is still employed in some court decisions. In *J.B. v. A.B.* (1978), a West Virginia case, both parents were deemed to be "fit" and the judge saw no other just means of deciding custody; therefore, he based his decision on the "tender years" doctrine. In *Fish v. Fish* (1968), an eight-year-old boy had been in his father's custody. The mother petitioned for custody and a lower court awarded the child to her on "tender years" stating that there was no substitute for motherly love. However, the Supreme Court ruled that the lower court could not explicitly base its decision solely on this tender years concept, and ruled in the father's favor, stating that the child and father had a close relationship. One should also note that the Supreme Court also took into consideration that a paternal grandmother was part of the family system, i.e., implicitly agreeing with the lower court that a surrogate mother is needed if custody is not awarded to the natural mother.

Implication for the Lesbian Mother

Although the tender years concept is not presently explicitly upheld in most cases, it is still implicitly recognized in many decisions.

The influence of the "tender years" concept may either help or hinder the lesbian mother's custody award depending on the judge's value system. If the judge feels that a child of "tender years" does not have an established sexual identity, the judge may feel the mother's lesbian lifestyle, values, and role modeling will have a negative effect upon the young child's development.

At the other end of the spectrum, the judge may be positively influenced toward award to the lesbian mother if the child is of "tender years" as in *Anderson v. Anderson* (Alexander, 1977), feeling that there is no substitute for motherly love whether she be heterosexual or homosexual. Although many states have technically dropped the "tender years" doctrine, no one is ever completely aware of all the factors that a court implicitly takes into account in making the final custody decisions.

Best Interests of Child

Until 1881, parental rights in child custody cases were primary. In *Chapsky v. Woods* (Alexander, 1977), Justice Brewer was the first to expound on the "best interests of the child." In 1925, in *Finlay v. Finlay,* Justice Cardoza reaffirmed this doctrine and under the Guardianship of Infants Act in the same year, mothers and fathers were given equal consideration for the custody of their children (Fine, 1980). Since that time many other concepts have been espoused in child custody cases, e.g., "tender year" and fitness, but the pendulum has swung back to the doctrine of the "best interests of the child."

In 1968 a Manifesto was put forth by the Uniform Child Custody Jurisdiction Act and adopted by the American Bar Association. The guidelines set down by the American Bar Association's

Family Law Section in 1973 viewed the concept of the best interests and welfare of the child as the primary consideration in custody, child support and visitation decisions. According to California Civil Code 4600, "The concept of custody embraces the combined interests of parents, the state and the child himself (Mills, p. 273). On reading this, one wonders, if the best interests of the child are primary, why is the child mentioned last? Some 21 states see the "best interests of the child" as residing with the natural parent unless this may be detrimental to the child (Smith, 1979).

The *Boyer v. Boyer* decision (Smith, 1979, p. 545) seems to sum up in ideal terms the interpretation of this concept: "when the child's right to a suitable custodian and the parent's rights are not in harmony, one must give way—and that is the parents' rights."

Anna Freud (Alexander, 1977) views the "best interests of the child" as encompassing three aspects—affection, stimulation, and unbroken continuity of affection. Each state varies on which aspect of the "best interest" doctrine it views as possessing the most weight in a child custody decision (Smith, 1979).

Implications for the Lesbian Mother

What constitutes the "best interest of the child" doctrine is vague and can be interpreted in a variety of ways. The concept may be interpreted in the mother's favor as per the traditional "tender years" doctrine (see ED. NOTE below).

In this instance, the lesbian mother would have priority over the father, if the judge did not consider sexual identity a factor. In contrast to this, the court may interpret the best interest of the child not to be served within a lesbian household *(Risher v. Risher,* Gibson, 1977). The concept is so vague and general, that it is possible for the judge and those he appoints, e.g., psychologist or guardian ad litem, to shape the concept interpretation to their own value system.

ED. NOTE: Admittedly the term "best interest of the child" is vague and indefinite. However, it must be noted this indefiniteness is the result of a deliberate legislative or legal decision designed to vest in the trial court the widest discretion to not only receive what is deemed evidence relevant to the issues of custody but also with respect to the ultimate issue of which parent is to be awarded custody.

There is no time frame mentioned in the concept; therefore, one can interpret it to mean future "best interests of the child. In the case of a lesbian mother, future predictions may be tenuous and unfavorable for her case. The "best interests of the child" may be served by awarding her custody at the present time, if she is not in a lesbian relationship. Five years from now, she may have set up household with another lesbian and the judge may feel that a stable lesbian household does fulfill the best interests of the child, as in *Schuster v. Schuster* (Beck, 1979).

If a judge considers the "best interests of the child" interpreted as moral or psychological interests, this might affect the award of custody to a lesbian mother. The determining factor is, where do the judge's priorities lie when considering "best interests of the child?" Is security more important than intellectual stimulation? Although the judge may ask for recommendations from the mental health field, it is the judge who has the power since that is where the final decision is made (some states have jury trials, e.g., Texas).

Although there seems to be some consensus about what is "bad" for a child, i.e., what is not in their best interests, there seems to be little agreement on what is in their "best interest." Since children develop so rapidly, physically and intellectually, what may be in their best interest at one point in time might be aversive to them at another phase of their development. In this light, the judge may consider the issue of sexual identity and role modeling as important. While it may not be an issue for the infant child of a lesbian mother at the time of the custody dispute, it may be an issue four years later.

The Principle of Continuity

Included in the "best interest of the child" concept is the idea of continuity, i.e., maintaining the child in the custodial home in which they have had an ongoing, stable relationship and environment.

In *Renflo v. Renflo* (Smith, 1979, p. 545), the court's opinion held that "continuity is probably the most important single element necessary to a child's wholesome development." Presently, eight states concur with this statement on child custody and maintain that continuity and stability are the primary factors to be considered in ascertaining the best interests of the child (Smith, 1979). Most courts and judges seem to feel that the maintenance of custody of the child with the parent who has had it up to this point is essential and that a child should never be transplanted unnecessarily (Jenkins, 1977).

Implications for the Lesbian Mother

If the continuity/stability concept is viewed in terms of the future, the lesbian mother, her attorney and expert witnesses may be faced with the dilemma of assuring or proving the stability of a lesbian relationship, if there is another woman involved. Although many lesbian relationships are tenuous, research shows that lesbians are more likely than male homosexuals to form dyadic and stable relationships (Tanner, 1978). In most lesbian mother custody cases (*Risher v. Risher*, Gibson, 1977; *Schuster v. Schuster*, Beck, 1979), the father's attorney was determined to prove the instability and ephemeral nature of the lesbian relationship.

If the judge defines continuity as evidenced in the lesbian mother's ongoing past relationship with her child, then some of the burden of proof is shifted to the father to prove otherwise. If the lesbian mother is able to demonstrate, through character witnesses, that her relationship with her child was constant and stable and that she is committed to having it remain that way she will have a better chance of being awarded custody. Witnesses, both expert and lay, are essential to the lesbian mother to show that she has maintained this type of environment for her child.

Support groups and other lesbian mothers admonish the lesbian mother involved in a child custody dispute against "copping out" at any point during the process, i.e., having her children stay elsewhere when the stress of the trial or process becomes overwhelming for her. Tremendous economic and psychological tensions besiege the lesbian mother who chooses to engage in a custody dispute, and she may feel it is best for both herself and her child to be separated to spare them grief and embarrassment. Since continuity receives such high priority, it seems that a separation at any point in time may jeopardize her chances of receiving custody.

The Decision to Fight

Many lesbian mothers never have to make the decision to fight for custody. They choose the option of "staying in the closet" or in the marriage for the sake of the children (Lewis, 1979). They not only hide their lesbianism from society, but many husbands and children are never confided in.

If she has concealed her lesbianism from her family and makes the decision to divorce and it is uncontested, her struggle to keep the children will be much easier. "By keeping silent about their lesbian feelings, they (lesbian mothers) manage to retain custody of their children" (Martin, 1972, p. 132). However, after obtaining custody, the lesbian mother then lives a precarious existence, besieged by the thoughts of her husband finding out later and seeking to modify the custody order, e.g., *Schuster v. Schuster* (Beck, 1979) or *Risher v. Risher* (Gibson, 1977).

If the lesbian mother has no option of revealing her lesbianism, i.e., her husband has found out or she has confided in him, then the struggle may begin. She has the option of fighting for her rights (?) or running from justice (?), i.e., kidnapping the children. Most cases involving lesbian mothers are settled out of court (Martin, 1972; Lewis, 1979). Support groups, such as NOW, the Lesbian Mothers' Union and the Lesbian Mothers' Defense Fund, urge lesbian mothers to avoid a custody showdown, if at all possible.

There are many issues that the lesbian mother has to resolve before the custody dispute begins. If her children have not already been told about her lesbianism, she must attempt to tell them at an age-appropriate level. Often relatives, friends, and co-workers must also be confided in since they may be needed as character witnesses.

If the custody is contested, the lesbian mother has another decision to make. Should she herself divulge her lesbianism to the court or should she force her husband to prove it? According to the decision in *Jordana v. Corley* (1975), if the mother has been awarded custody and the father, on discovering she is a lesbian seeks to modify or change the custody order, the burden of proof rests on the person seeking the change to show that the change in custody is essential in protecting the child's welfare. It is possible for the lesbian mother and her attorney to introduce a motion to bar the issue of homosexuality from the record. Often this request is denied (*Risher v. Risher,* Gibson, 1977).

Why would a lesbian mother choose to fight? Often she has no other option since her lesbianism is public knowledge. For some lesbian mothers, it is a "cause." When she is embroiled in battle, the lesbian mother discovers in whom her support systems and trust lie. She is in a very vulnerable position, economically and psychologically. She is often forced to take a temporary leave of absence from her job *(Risher v. Risher,* Gibson, 1977) to prepare her defense and to de-emphasize her place of employment in the media. Capable and recognized expert witnesses need to be chosen by her attorney. It is often difficult to find expert witnesses willing to become involved in the struggle. Usually support groups can provide referrals. NOW supports test cases referred to the Lesbian Mothers' Defense Fund, although they encourage the lesbian mother to pursue all other avenues before fighting for custody (Vida, 1978).

There are cases of husbands becoming involved in contesting custody cases and then withdrawing the petitions. This manipulation often provides him with alimony or child support on his terms (Kirschner, 1979).

The Winners (?)

What personal characteristics and factors assist the lesbian mother in child custody disputes? In most cases in which the lesbian mother was awarded custody, she had been married for a number of years, was well-known in the community and respected, was older (over 35), and her children were not of "tender years," i.e., their sexual identity was established (Martin, 1972).

It is believed by some attorneys and expert witnesses that it also helps if the children of a lesbian mother are males *(Risher v. Risher,* Gibson, 1977). If the children are females and the mother is living with a lover, there is then the perceived possibility that either the mother or the lover might at some point seduce the female child.

The Losers

In *Risher v. Risher* (Gibson, 1977), Mary Jo Risher, a 36-year-old lesbian mother of two boys (16 and 7 years old) was fighting for custody of her younger son. Her attorney thought that many things were in her favor, e.g., she was 36 years old, had been a nurse for a number of years, had been married for sixteen years in a stable and committed relationship. Many things, however, were not in her favor, e.g., she was living with a lover and her son was of "tender years." Her husband had remarried and now wanted custody of both boys. In many cases *(Schuster v. Schuster,* Beck, 1979), as in this one, the ex-husband did not acknowledge a desire to have custody until he remarried. In the case of *Risher v. Risher* (Gibson, 1977), the ex-husband had had a vasectomy and could not have any more children. If the ex-husband sees the wife's lesbianism as an attack to his male ego, much anger may be vented by and through the custody dispute. The general reaction of these ex-husbands towards their ex-spouses is, "I'll show the world what you are" (Gibson, 1977, p. 147).

A child custody dispute is usually held in domestic relations or family court and seldom goes before a jury. One of the exceptions to this is in the state of Texas, where a jury trial is still held for a custody battle. *Risher v. Risher* (Gibson, 1977) was the first known jury trial involving the custody rights of a lesbian mother. The jurors were composed of 10 males and 2 females with supposedly no prejudice against homosexuals or no knowledge of the homosexual lifestyles. Mary Jo Risher was physically, emotionally and economically drained through the court battle for custody. After spending thousands of dollars and thousands of hours of precious time, custody was awarded to her husband. At the writing of her book (Gibson, 1977), Mary Jo Risher was appealing the decision which she estimated would cost her another $5,000 (see ED. NOTE following).

ED. NOTE: This paper has been included in this volume because it discusses a unique issue concerning custody of children which the therapist may encounter, i.e., children of gay parents (see Riddle and Arguelles, "Children of Gay Parents: Homophobia's Victims," in *Children of Separation and Divorce,* edited by Stuart and Abt, 1981). If one concedes, as we believe we must, that ethics and law parallel the general mores of society, the premise of this chapter is correct that, as opposed to a custody dispute between otherwise competent parents, the gay parent who seeks custody of children is at a disadvantage when opposed by the normal parent. Society's views of the homosexual, historically and currently, are too well-known to need recounting here. Suffice it to say, homosexual behavior has been and still is viewed as perverted, pathological, immoral and sinful. Those states using concepts of "fitness" to determine custody issues have little or no difficulty in determining the gay parent to be "unfit." Those states applying "best interest of the child" standards, also generally have little difficulty in determining that the best interest of the child is better served by being raised in what society views as a normal environment. There will always be concern the child may be turned into a homosexual, deprived of a normal childhood and upbringing, and improperly prepared for adulthood. Riddle and Arguelles point out the unique stresses imposed upon the child of a gay parent and of opportunities for the child to

REFERENCES

Abbott, S. & Love, B. *Sappho was a right on woman.* NY: Stein & Day, 1972.

Alexander, S. Protecting the child's rights in custody cases, *Family Coordinator,* 1977, *26*(4), 377–382.

Beck, P. Nontraditional life styles, *Journal of Family Law,* 1979, *17*(4), 685–710.

Benedek, R. & Benedek, E. The child's preference in Michigan custody disputes, *American Journal of Family Therapy,* 1979, *2*(4), 37–43.

Druckman, J. & Rhodes, C. Family impact analysis: Application to child custody determination, *Family Coordinator,* 1977, *26*(14), 451–458.

Ferleger, D. The battles over children's rights, *Social Issues: 1979–80,* Connecticut: Dushkin Publishing Groups, Inc., 1979, 230–232.

Gibson, G. *By her own admission,* NY: Doubleday & Co., 1977.

Jenkins, R. Maxims in child custody cases, *Family Coordinator,* 1977, *26*(4), 385–389.

Kenney, E., Chambers, W., & Rodman, W. *Law of California Relating to Women and Children.* California: Baumgardt Publishing Co., 1978.

Kingdon, M. Lesbians, *Counseling Psychologist,* 1979, *8*(1), 44–45.

Kirschner, S. Child Custody determination: A better way, *Journal of Family Law,* 1979, *17*(2), 275–296.

Levin, H. & Askin, F. Privacy in the courts: Law and social reality, *Journal of Social Issues,* 1977, *33*(3), 138–152.

Lewis, S. *Sunday's Women.* Boston: Beacon Press, 1979.

McFadden, M. *Bachelor Fatherhood,* NY: Grosset & Dunlap, 1974.

Martin, D. & Lynn, P. *Lesbian Woman.* San Francisco: Glide Publishers, 1972.

Mills, B. Custody in California, in *The Family Law Symposium,* Los Angeles Superior Court, 295, 303, 1979.

Mnookin, R. Child custody adjudication: Judicial function in the face of indeterminacy, *Law and Contemporary Problems,* 1975, *39*(3), 226–293.

---

manipulate the closet homosexual parent. Both events are not conducive to the longterm best interest of the child. The Riddle-Arguelles study disclosed that 79% of their sample of 164 children lived with the gay parent. If the mother was a lesbian, the chances were 58% of living with that parent. If the gay parent was male, the child's chance was 21%, and 69% of the sample were in the legal custody of the gay parent. This study would seem to indicate that perhaps the legal system when compelled to deal with children of gay parents is not so biased as suggested. See also Mills, 1979 and his discussion of "Homosexuality of the parent as a factor in the determination of custody," at 300, 301. ED: DBH.

Morin, S. & Schultz, S. The Gay Movement and the rights of children, *Journal of Social Issues,* 1978, *34*(2), 137–148.

Musetto, A. Child custody and visitation: The role of the clinician in relation to the family, *Family Therapy,* 1978, *5*(2), 143–150.

Pred, E. (Ed.). Studies & Surveys, *The Advocate,* May 31, 1978.

Riddle, D. Relating to children: Gays as role models, *Journal of Social Issues,* 1978, *34*(3), 34–54.

Sagarin, E. The high personal cost of wearing a label, *Social Issues: 1979–80,* Connecticut: Dushkin Publishing Group, Inc., 1979.

Shilts, R. Lesbian Mothers' Defense Funds: Apple Pie Battles, *The Advocate,* October 22, 1978.

Smith, S. Psychological parent vs. biological parent: The court's response to new directions in child custody dispute resolution, *Journal of Family Law,* 1979, *17*(3), 545–576.

Snyder, P. & Martin, L. Leaving the family out of family court: Criminalizing the juvenile justice system, *American Journal of Orthopsychiatry,* 1978, *48*(3), 390–393.

Tanner, D. *The Lesbian Couple,* Massachusetts: D. C. Heath & Co., 1978.

Vida, G. *Our Right to Love,* N.J.: Prentice Hall, Inc., 1978.

Weiss, W. & Collada, H. Conciliation counseling: The Courts effective mechanism for resolving visitation and custody disputes, *Family Coordinator,* 1977, *26*(4), 444–450.

Fine, S. Children of divorce, custody and access situations: The contribution of the mental health professional, *Journal of Counseling Psychology & Psychiatry,* 1980, *21*(4), 353–361.

Woody, R. Fathers with child custody, *The Counseling Psychologist,* 1978, *7*(4), 60–63.

Wysor, B. *The Lesbian Myth,* NY: Random House, 1974.

Zelkind, S. Civil liberties: an overview of some contributions from the behavioral sciences, *Journal of Social Issues,* 1975, *31*(2), 138–152.

CASES CITED

J. B. v. A. B., W. Va. 242 S. E. 2d 248 (1978).

Schall v. Schall, Pa. Super., 380 A. 2d 478 (1977).

McGowan v. McGowan, Pa. Super., 374 A. 2d 1306 (1977).

Bennett v. Jeffreys, 40 N. Y. 2d 543, 356 N. E. 2d 277 (1976).

Schuster v. Schuster, 90 Wash. 2d 626, 585 P. 2d 130 (1978).

Stanley v. Illinois, 405 U. S. 645 (1972).

The Ethical, Legal and Pragmatic Issues of Sexual Countertransference and Sex Therapy

CHAPTER 7

LAUREL BONHAM-DUVALL

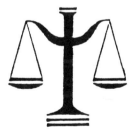

THE ETHICAL, LEGAL AND PRAGMATIC ISSUES OF SEXUAL COUNTERTRANSFERENCE AND SEX THERAPY

7

Laurel Bonham-Duvall

Principle 6 of the *Ethical Standards of Psychologists* (1979, p.5) makes it clear that "sexual intimacies with clients are unethical." This statement echoes the sentiments of Sigmund Freud, who believed that sexual relations with clients would destroy the analytic relationship and would be an excuse for undermining the reputation and professionalism of psychology (Dahlberg, 1970). Most therapists publicly agree with this ethic, recognizing the potential for exploitation of their clients if they were to succumb to temptation.

However, the literature has revealed a growing and popular underground movement for legitimizing sexual relations in therapy within the last twenty years. This movement was shockingly revealed by McCartney in 1966 in an article called "Overt Transference." McCartney expressly named several leading psychologists who advocated and practiced sex in therapy, including Wilhelm Reich and Ernest Jones. McCartney was chastised by his peers as unethical (Kardener, Fuller, & Mensh, 1973).

McCartney's article was paralleled by the revelations of the work by Masters and Johnson (1966) which included behavioral methods of treating sexual dysfunctions. In Masters and Johnson's therapy, if one did not have a partner, they provided a "surrogate therapist" (Leroy, 1972; Greene, 1977) who would do "bodywork" (Greene, 1977) with the client. The world waited breathlessly for charges of prostitution and exploitation but they never came. Instead that clinic and its sex therapy were applauded and used as a model across the country (Leroy, 1972).

In the 1977s a number of investigators (Kardener, et al., 1973; Butler & Zelen, 1977) conducted surveys of the incidence of "erotic behavior" utilized by psychologists, psychiatrists, and other physicians. Kardener and associates found that five percent of their sample had engaged in erotic contact although few had actually had intercourse, whereas in 1977, Butler and Zelen estimated that 20 percent were "intimate" with their clients. Both research groups reported that the primary reason for erotic behavior was due to uncontrolled countertransference by needy, vulnerable, or lonely therapists, rather than for patients' best interests. These studies and one done by Dahlberg (1970) found that most of the therapists who sexually acted out were males over forty who were having difficulties with their marriages at that time or who were separated or divorced. Their clients were typically younger females.

These studies tend to reinforce the image of the "dirty old man" in middle-age crisis who uses his position and power in the therapeutic situation to seduce his needy and vulnerable client into bed to satisfy his own lust. This image may be real as the many court cases discussed in this chapter seem to indicate. The traditional solution has been to have the therapist go into analysis so that he may know himself well enough to be able to avoid problems in countertransference; that is, the projection of emotions or attributes onto the patient (Dahlberg, 1970; Chaplin, 1968). Countertransference has been seen as a hindrance since Freud's time because of the possible danger of being consciously or unconsciously compromised (Dahlberg, 1970; Epstein & Feiner, 1979). The APA Ethics Committee (1979) still views analysis as the best recourse for violation of ethics.

Current theorists who are concerned about countertransference no longer see countertransference as a hinderance (Dunn & Dickes, 1977; Marshall, 1979); nor is it as simple as once believed (Dahlberg, 1970; Epstein & Feiner, 1979).

Field theory has illuminated the fact that the therapist-client interaction is a very complex interaction of projections, associations and responses (Marshall, 1979). As Freud once sketchily hypothesized, countertransference is a combination of the therapist's own internal emotions, thoughts and behaviors as well as the reception of the clients' conscious or unconscious emotions (Marshall, 1979). Therapists may or may not be aware of the emotions they are receiving and sending, nor may the client. However, unclear and unanalyzed interactions, especially those involving resistances, can lead to some form of withdrawal from the interaction or even to sudden sexual or aggressive acting out (Dickes & Strauss, 1979; Epstein & Feiner, 1979; Marshall, 1979).

There is a controversy over whether or not to discuss interactions pertaining to sexual attraction countertransferences, however. Some therapists believe such discussion will heighten sexual arousal and actually lead to acting out (Ulanov, 1979; Dahlberg, 1970; McCartney, 1966; Greene, 1977). Others believe that analyzing the interaction will get to the issues behind the sexual feelings and thereby defuse the situation (Marshall, 1979; Ulanov, 1979; Epstein & Feiner, 1979; Dahlberg, 1970; Levay, Kagle, & Weissberg, 1979; Will, 1979; Fordham, 1979; Grey, 1979). All seem to agree, however, that countertransference emotions are the key to understanding the internal processes of the client.

The question of whether to discuss sexual attraction or not is very important. There is danger that discussion of sexual attraction may lead to acting out if there is a strong attraction already. If the situation is not handled carefully, all therapeutic benefit can be lost. On the other hand, if sexual attraction is an issue and it is avoided, there may be no therapeutic benefit at all. In both instances, most theorists would agree that the therapist as well as the client lose. According to APA, it is better to refer the client out or terminate therapy than to risk acting out (American Psychological Association, 1979).

Butler and Zelen (1977) provide a good example of the predicament from an interview question that they asked 20 therapists who had had sex with clients:

> How did sexual contact develop and what sort of rationalizations were used? In most cases the therapist, in his leadership role, would bring up the issue of his sexual attraction to the patient. In many cases, the patient responded favorably to these innuendoes. Subsequently, there was an acceptance of the mutuality of this attraction and somehow, vaguely, the therapist lost control of the therapeutic hour. . . In some situations the therapists' innuendoes led to further discussion of the mutual attraction, and then resulted in intercourse (Buttler & Zelen, 1977, 141-142).

McCartney (1966) and Reich (1949) would disagree that therapeutic goals are lost when sex occurs in therapy. They believed that genital excitation reactivates the original sexual conflict between parents and child and allows a reworking of this conflict in therapy. McCartney claimed that by allowing full sexual expression within the therapeutic alliance (not a social relationship), the client will be able to work through the conflict and mature rather than become frustrated and regress again. McCartney quoted Reich (1949) as saying:

> The important thing is that in this process they learn to tolerate genital frustration, that for the first time they do not react with disappointment, and they do not regress. They concentrate both emotional and somatic strivings on the analyst. Patients who fail to go through such Overt Transference of a genital character do not succeed in fully establishing genital primacy. In such cases, the analyst has either not succeeded in really liberating from repression the sexual strivings, or he has not succeeded in dissolving the guilt feelings (McCartney, 1966, p.230).

McCartney suggests that so long as persons are unable to have a successful sexual experience, their chances of having a mature sexual relationship are limited. Those who are mature enough to find a mate outside of the therapeutic relationship will find one; those who are unable to find one will need the therapist's help before they can succeed in establishing a heterosexual relationship.

Without a thorough examination of McCartney's article, his ideas seem extremely liberal, even bizarre. However, he seems to be saying what Masters and Johnson have advocated: that the single, sexually dysfunctional person has the right to therapeutic treatment of their dysfunctions, whether they be physical or psychological (Leroy, 1972).

It has been said that a sexually dysfunctional male is "a societal cripple," and that one might ask, "Does society want them treated?. . . If they are not treated it is discrimination of one segment of society over another" (from *Time*, May 25, 1970, p. 49, quoted in Leroy, 1972).

Such a philosophy gives some insight into the attitudes of those few members of Kardener's (1973) and Butler and Zelen's (1977) samples who believed that they had had sex with their clients for the patients' "best interests." Kardener and associates seemed surprised by the 13 percent of their sample who described circumstances in which they believed that sex or erotic contact with clients might have been helpful, although few of that 13 percent had actually had contact with their patients.

Such behavior might be useful, they suggested, in treating sexual maladjustments, depression in middle-aged women who feel undesirable, specific sexual problems, and sexual frustration in widows and divorcees. They also listed other areas in which erotic contact might be helpful: increasing clients' self-esteem through recognition of their sexual status, in disclosing areas of sexual blocking, in demonstrating no physical cause for absence of libido, in allowing the expression of sex in mature patients flowing with nonconflicted [love] feelings, and in "making therapy go further and deeper" (Karden, et al., 1973, p. 1079). Some of these suggestions were made by physicians, but most were made by psychiatrists.

What Kardener and associates and McCartney (1966), as well as Masters and Johnson, are implying is that there are circumstances in our society where clients are unable to establish relationships, for whatever reason, that satisfy their needs for creature comfort or sex. Consciously or unconsciously, clients may bring these needs into the therapy relationship and express these needs via the transference relationship. Depending on the state of the therapist in his own life, the purpose of the therapy, and the competence of the therapist to defuse the situation, sexual acting-out could occur. The therapist's subsequent reaction to the situation could be therapeutic, or could lead to hurt, anger, frustration, guilt, or embarrassment for both client and therapist, and potential damage to the patient, a lawsuit and/or loss of licensure for the therapist. The laws and ethics to date do not recognize the potential for legitimate use of sex between therapist and client in therapy (Sherwin, 1966; Leroy, 1972).

The laws that can come into play in a sexual relationship fall under the general categories of malpractice, moral turpitude, undue influence, prostitution/pimping/pandering, unprofessional opportunism, negligence, rape, adultery, fornication, or other criminal or civil charges (Schwitzgebel & Schwitzgebel, 1980; Perr, 1975). Punishments can consist of fines, probation, revocation of licensure, or imprisonment, depending on the charge and circumstances. Since most cases are handled in the lower trial courts and seldom reach Appellate Court, there are only a handful of cases for which the results are recorded (Sherwin, 1966). There are hundreds of malpractice suits each year that are not recorded (Butler & Zelen, 1977).

The major cases which deal with the mishandling of the countertransference dilemma include: *Landau v. Werner; Colorado*

State Board of Medical Examiners v. Weiler; Bernstein v. Board of Medical Examiners; Zipkin v. Freeman; Anclote Manor Foundation v. Wilkinson; Whitesell v. Green; Morra v. State Board of Examiners of Psychologists; and Roys v. Hartogs (Perr, 1975; Schwitzgebel (Schwitzgebel, 1980).

In *Landau v. Weiner* (1961) the court decided that the therapist should have referred the patient elsewhere as instructed by the APA ethics, as soon as he had "fallen in love." The *Weiler* case considered the therapists' recommendation of extramarital intercourse and the filling of that prescription himself to be "grossly negligent malpractice" (1965). *Bernstein* (1962) was charged and found guilty of statutory rape of a 16-year old girl, in spite of the pretext of medical treatment (See ED. NOTE below.)

In *Zipkin v. Freeman*, the charge was a mishandling of the transference relationship (Perr, 1975), but this case was considered to be more than an abuse of a professional relationship. In concurring with the decision, Judge Eager stated:

> Regardless of all psychiatric theories, whether of transference, withdrawal, or otherwise, this relationship (and the doctor's acts) passed the point at which anyone could logically believe that they had any reasonable connection with professional services, or that they were being performed in the course of any legitimate treatment. In other words, the "treatment" ceased, and an ordinary, person-to-person, invasion of plaintiff's rights . . . began. . . . one does not conduct an illicit adventure with a woman over a period of months through negligence, professional or otherwise (436 S.W. 2d 753, 1968, in Perr, 1975, p.38).

The *Anclote Manor Foundation v. Wilkinson* case concerned a psychiatrist who again overstepped his ethical boundary in countertransference by allegedly telling his patient that he would marry her. The charge was for breach of contract in providing psychiatric and medical services. The psychiatrist "destroyed the possibility of benefit that could have been anticipated under skillful treatment" (Perr, 1975, p.38).

ED. NOTE: This case, involving as it did a minor, demonstrates also the need for parental or court consent to what may be considered unusual therapy techniques. However, intercourse with an underaged female is a criminal act the parents may not consent to.

In *Whitesell v. Green* (1973), the psychologist was found to be legally liable for having had an affair with his patient's wife, even though he claimed he had terminated his professional relationship with the patient two weeks prior to the sexual relationship with the wife (Schwitzgebel & Schwitzgebel, 1980). This is an interesting case, since ethically, according to APA Principle 2, the psychologist had the duty to terminate the case (as he did) or refer it, and then had the option of pursuing the relationship. It would seem then that he would have mainly been liable for adultery. However, more information would be needed to clarify the issues in this case.

In the *Morra* case, the court upheld the decision by the state licensing agency to revoke Morra's license for having sex with two patients. "The board had found the psychologist's actions to be negligent and wrongful. It said he he had ignored a basic duty of a responsible psychologist—to avoid sexual intimacies with his patients—and had failed to consider his patient's well-being" (Perr, 1975, p.37).

More recently, in *Roys v. Hartogs*, a psychiatrist allegedly contracted with a woman to cure her lesbianism by "administering" sexual intercourse to her. Schwitzgebel and Schwitzgebel (1980) discussed this case, stating:

> The patient claimed that she was coerced into having sexual relations because of his overpowering influence and her reasonable trust in his competency. The court remanded the matter to a jury, stating that because the plaintiff consulted the defendant about sexual problems, the treatment prescribed was not palpably unreasonable and thereby might induce a patient to submit to sexual relations. The trial court assessed $25,000 in punitive damages. A dissenting judge noted, however, that the patient was capable of giving consent and did not complain until after the relationship was terminated. . . . Although consent does not mitigate liability for malpractice it may act as a defense against claim of deception, fraud, or battery (cited in 381 N.Y.S. 2d 587, 591. SupCt. Appl. Ter., 1976, in Schwitzgebel & Schwitzgebel, 1980, p.256).

The psychotherapist enjoys the trust and confidence of his patients which enables the psychotherapist to influence the patient. Thus the psychotherapist is peculiarly able to take advantage of the relationship to the detriment of the patient. As the cases discussed above demonstrate, the courts and state licensing agencies act to protect clients from being taken advantage of by therapists who use their positions of influence and power to satiate their own needs and desires, rather than to work for the best interests of the clients.

In Schwitzbegel and Schwitzgebel's (1980) notes, a quote by Dawidoff (p.265, Note 58) suggests that if clients feel that sex is in their own best interest and the therapist agrees, then, "intimacies of the psychiatrist/patient relationship may be all right so long as the patient remains the initiator." The judges in the *Hartogs* case also seemed to be implying that as long as the client gives "informed consent," the therapist may have a defense. The problem is that in a countertransference relationship, it is difficult to tell who was the actual initiator and what consequences may occur in the relationship. It is up to individual therapists to know themselves well enough to be able to know what they would do in various circumstances, keeping in mind that the courts, juries, and state licensing agencies will not be sympathetic.

It is significant that "not a single criminal prosecution of a sex clinic participant has been called... to attention" (Leroy, 1972, p.594). Leroy (1972) claimed that Masters and Johnson's surrogates could have been charged with prostitution, and that Masters and Johnson and their foundation with pimping, pandering and procuring, and their clients for soliciting, loitering in a house of prostitution, patronizing or aiding and abetting prostitution. While the claim may be hyperbole, it represents a still pervasive attitude concerning sex in the therapeutic relationship.

Although many of the sexual and prostitution laws are out-of-date and unenforced (Sherwin, 1966), the legislative intent of prostitution laws, are, according to Leroy:

- To prevent all sex activity between any person other than spouse (or consenting adults in California and Illinois)
- To prevent the sexual and economic exploitation of women by police, men, and disease
- To control the spread of venereal disease
- To further the rehabilitation of fallen women
- To protect the civic reputation by projecting a low image of vice and corruption (Leroy, 1972, p.600)

Leroy also suggested that the reason that Masters and Johnson and their colleagues have avoided prosecution has been their cultivation of public opinion and their strict adherence to "medical" goals, methods, and terminology. He stated:

An effective treatment clinic would not frustrate the achievement of these goals [as stated above], and might in some ways help attain them. Since the surrogate program is medically oriented and supervised, its women certainly will not be exploited by disease. . . Because the female therapists are screened to be feminine, resourceful, well-adjusted, and therefore effective in treating both physical and mental problems, it is doubtful that a program will create either "fallen women" or much sexual or economic exploitation. . . Since the public contact of the therapist and patient assumes the appearance of ordinary social dating, and as all other contacts are made in private, the surrogate programs present no highly visible public eyesore. . ." (Leroy, 1972, p.600).

Although the judges' comments in the *Roys v. Hartogs* case seem to support the above statement by Leroy, the verdict of the jury shattered the security which therapists who advocate behavioral sex therapy treatments might feel. Obviously, the public was not ready for such ideas. However, each case is different and it is the intent and purpose of the therapy which is important. If the therapist's intent in "administering" sex is *indisputably* for the welfare of the patient, then the treatment may be permissable by law. Here, Principle 6 of the Ethical Standards of Psychologists is applicable:

Psychologists are continually cognizant of their own needs and of their inherently powerful position *vis a vis* clients, in order to avoid exploiting their trust and dependency. Psychologists make every effort to avoid dual relationships which might impair their professional judgment or increase the risk of client exploitation. Sexual intimacies with clients are unethical (American Psychological Association, 1979, p. 5).

Dual relationships refer to having two types of relationships with one person, one therapeutic and one social. If a therapist falls in love or wants to see a client socially, he should refer the patient elsewhere for treatment, as suggested in the *Landau* case. Butler and Zelen (1977) found that although most of their subjects in their research knew of this obligation, few actually did, presumably due to fear of exposure, embarrassment or denial. By not following this principle, they and others like them risk grave embarrassment, plus loss of money, license, or liberty. The precept of APA Principle 6 is that there is no legitimate use of sex in therapy when the sex is between the psychotherapist and patient (American Psychological Association, 1979, p.2).

Principle 3, pertaining to Moral and Legal Standards, suggests that psychologists conform their personal moral, ethical and legal standards of behavior to those of the prevailing community if their behavior may "compromise the fulfillment of their professional responsibilities, or reduce the trust in psychology or psychologists held by the general public" (American Psychological Association, 1979, p.2).

It is crucial that the client is competent and gives voluntary and *informed* consent about any treatment that is given—sexual or otherwise. In sex therapy, this includes informing the client of the possibility of mishandling the countertransference; or if behavioral sexual techniques are used, informing the client of what might occur during the treatment and as a result of the treatment; for example, that the client may feel hurt, damaged or abused. Such consent should preferably be all in writing. This precaution will help insure a trusting, open, and more egalitarian relationship, thus minimizing the threat of undue influence. It may also prevent an otherwise potentially harmful relationship from developing. However, remember that Schwitzgebel and Schwitzgebel (1980, p.256) stated "consent does not mitigate liability for malpractice. . ." and in most states sex between the therapist and the patient is not only unethical, it constitutes possible malpractice.

Nonjudgmental peer support groups and supervision during times of stress or with potentially incendiary relationships are desperately needed in order to help therapists avoid problems or to handle them effectively. Those therapists who have personal problems should be helped to recognize them and they should be kept from doing therapy where sexual techniques are used.

It is important that sex therapists continue to educate and inform the public of the purposes of sex in therapy. They should advocate that laws and ethics should be changed or restated to protect their profession as well as safeguard the clients. Sex therapists must also take extra precautions to prevent quackery from infiltrating the field and violating the tenuous trust between the public and sex clinics. This means helping the public and fellow therapists define the difference between professional use of sexual techniques and overstepping the bounds of countertransference into dual relationships.

REFERENCES

American Psychological Association, *Ethical Standards of Psychologists,* 1979.

Butler, S. & Zelen, S. Sexual intimacies between therapists and patients, *Psychotherapy: Theory, Research and Practice, 14*(2), 1977, 139–145.

Chaplin, J. *Dictionary of Psychology,* NY: Dell Publishing Co., Inc., 1968.

Dahlberg, C. Sexual contact between patient and therapist, *Contemporary Psychoanalysis, 7,* 1970, 107–114.

Dickes, R. & Strauss, D. Countertransference as a factor in premature termination of apparently successful cases, *Journal of Sex and Marital Therapy, 5*(1), 1979, 22–27.

Dunn, M. & Dickes, R. Erotic issues in cotherapy, *Journal of Sex and Marital Therapy, 3*(3), 1977, 205–211.

Epstein, L. & Feiner, A. Countertransference: The therapists's contribution to treatment, *Contemporary Psychoanalysis, 15*(3), 1979, 489–513.

Fordham, M. Analytical psychology and countertransference, *Contemporary Psychoanalysis, 15*(4), 1979, 630–646.

Greene, S. Resisting the pressure to become a surrogate: A case study, *Journal of Sex and Marital Therapy, 3*(1), 1977, 40–49.

Grey, A. Countertransference and parataxis, *Contemporary Psychoanalysis, 15*(3), 1979, 472–483.

Kardener, S., Fuller, M., & Mensh, I. Survey of physician's attitudes and practices regarding erotic and nonerotic contact with patients, *American Journal of Psychiatry, 130*(10), 1973, 1077–1081.

Leroy, D. The potential criminal liability of human sex clinics and their patients, *Saint Louis University Law Journal, 16,* 1972, 586–603.

Levay, A., Kagle, A., & Weissberg, J. Issues of transference in sex therapy, *Journal of Sex and Marital Therapy, 5*(1), 1979, 15–21.

Marshall, R. Countertransference in the psychotherapy of children and adolescents, *Contemporary Psychoanalysis, 15*(4), 1979, 595–629.

McCartney, J. Overt transference, *Journal of Sex Research, 2*(3), 1966, 227–237.

McCarthy, B. Strategies and techniques for the reduction of sexual anxiety, *Journal of Sex and Marital Therapy, 3*(4), 1977, 243–248.

Mosher, D. The Gestalt awareness-expression cycle as a model for sex therapy, *Journal of Sex and Marital Therapy, 3*(4), 1977, 229–242.

Perr, I. Legal aspects of sexual therapies, *The Journal of Legal Medicine, 3,* 1975, 33–38.

Schwitzgebel, R. & Schwitzgebel, R. *Law and Psychological Practice*, NY: John Wiley & Sons, 1980.

Sherwin, R. The law and sexual relationships, *Journal of Social Issues, 22,* 1966, 109–122.

Ulanov, A. Follow-up treatment in cases of patient/therapist sex, *Journal of the American Academy of Psychoanalysis, 7*(1), 101–110.

Will, O., Jr. Comments on the professional life of the psychotherapist, *Contemporary Psychoanalysis, 15*(40), 560–576.

Wilson, G. Ethical and professional issues in sex therapy: Comments on Bailey's "Psychotherapy or massage parlor technology?" *Journal of Consulting and Clinical Psychology, 46*(6), 1978, 1510–1514.

LEGAL CASES (Cited either in Schwitzgebel & Schwitzgebel, 1980, or Perr, 1975).

Anclote Manor Foundation v. Wilkinson, Fla., 263 So.2d 256 (1972).

Bernstein v. Board of Medical Examiners, 204 C.A.2d 378, 22 Cal. Rptr. 419 (1962).

Colorado State Board of Medical Examiners v. Weiler, 157 Col. 244, 402 P.2d 606 (1965).

Landau v. Werner, 105 Solicitor's Journal 1008 (1961).

Morra v. State Board of Examiners of Psychologists, 212 Kan. 103, 510 P.2d 614 (1973).

Roys v. Hartogs, 366 N.Y.S.2d 297 (N.Y.C. Civ. Ct. 1975).

Whitesell v. Green, Hawaii Dist. Ct., Honolulu, Docket No. 38745, Nov. 19, 1973; reported in 28 CITATION 172.

Zipkin v. Freeman, 436 S.W.2d 753 (1968).

To Love Or Not To Love?
That Is The Question

CHAPTER 8

MARIE HEWETT

TO LOVE OR NOT TO LOVE? THAT IS THE QUESTION

Marie Hewett

I seldom write papers from a subjective stance. This however will be one of those rare occasions when I do since it has become apparent to me that ethics are indeed a highly personal matter, and it is only, in the final analysis, my own values, feelings and actions that are relevant in this arena.

In other words, I can only speak for myself. Furthermore, I doubt that this paper will generate any original or novel ideas. More than anything else, what I expect it will do is to increase and structure my own knowledge of the topic area and thereby provide a basis from which I can operate, should the need ever arise.

I've often wondered what I would do if I were to find myself in love with a client and that client in love with me. I'm fully aware that many people who seek counseling are not "sick"—some are totally delightful, intelligent, good human beings who, for some reason, have reached an impasse in their lives. I'm also quite aware that, aside from my professional status, I am only human. Like everyone else, I have needs and feelings. And, like most folks, I do fall in love now and then. I am not emotionally infallible or invulnerable.

Much has been written about transference and countertransference, most of it from an impersonal and objective standpoint, with the bulk of the literature on the subject originating from the psychoanalytic school of thought, and most of those holding other theoretical viewpoints treating the concepts rather casually and/or superficially. Even definitions of transference and countertransference show a great deal of variability. In its most general sense, transference refers to any feelings (whether a rational reaction to the person of the therapist or the unconscious projection of earlier attitudes and stereotypes) a client may feel or express toward the therapist, while countertransference refers to feelings, real or projected, the therapist experiences in regard to the client (Brammer & Shostrom, 1977). Psychoanalysts take a very rigid view of the concepts, seeing transference as a total projection process on the part of the client and countertransference as a problem to be dealt with (eliminated) by the therapist via supervision and personal psychotherapy (Hendrick, 1968; Tarachow, 1963; Goldman & Milman, 1978; Blanck, 1976). At the more liberal end of the spectrum are those who feel that clinical definitions of transference and countertransference serve to unduly intellectualize and externalize what is really a very personal relationship, and that feelings felt by either the client or the therapist are normal and should therefore not be considered disturbing or pathological (Brammer & Shostrom, 1977; Polster & Polster, 1974).

My own orientation tends toward the latter point of view, since I feel that a large part of successful psychotherapy is based on providing the client with a corrective emotional and interpersonal relationship, in addition to enhancing awareness, fostering insight and facilitating adaptive behaviors.

And I don't see how anyone can do that without feeling *something*! Indeed, I'm sure almost all theoreticians would acknowledge that some amount of transference exists in every therapeutic relationship, as does countertransference, since for interpersonal interaction there must be at least a modicum of emotional involvement. Without it there could only be flat indifference. Since emotions do not exist in isolation but are instead not unlike a magnetic field between people (May, 1969), transference and countertransference might be seen as somewhat reciprocal processes, to varying extents, and as being mutually reinforcing (Goldman & Milman, 1978). To be sure, I've had my own countertransference experiences—anger, boredom, irritation, frustration.

I have liked some clients more than I have others, just as I like some of my friends (or instructors, classmates, pets, acquaintances, relatives) more than I do others. I am, after all, only human. And I am sure these very ordinary and human emotional reactions are a blend of both realistic and unconscious (transference) components.

Romantic love. It would seem to me that this phenomenon has perhaps more than anything else, the potential for incorporating a great deal of transference. In fact I would suspect it is entirely possible that two people who are madly in love with one another are, for the most part, engaging in a massive transference exchange.

Fromme (1965) defined romantic love as a projection process, a being in love with love, being in love with one's own creation. He indicated that it was characterized by self-centeredness, impulsiveness, excesses, irrationality and impermanence; that it represented a perfect flight from intelligence and reason; and that it incorporated vast quantities of idealization of the other. (Yes, that does maybe sound like transference. . . .)

Reik (1963) indicated that we all have a need to be loved; that people do not live in a social vacuum; that human beings are social creatures; that every individual needs love, recognition, and affection; that we feel happy when the wishes of our childhood—for unconditional love and acceptance—*seem* to come true. (That perhaps sounds like transference too. . . .)

Peele (1975) took the concept a step further, seeing addictive (romantic) love as a form of dependency, not unlike dependency on (addiction to) other externals, such as alcohol, drugs, tobacco, and food.

I'm personally inclined to think that no one's dependency needs are ever entirely and perfectly met during childhood, so that the need for and the susceptibility to romantic love—that much-touted and epitomized transference phenomenon of our era—exists along a continuum of intensity rather than as an "either-or" concept.

Meissner (1978) was essentially in agreement with the aforementioned authors, seeing lack of individuation, poor self-boundaries, fragile self-identity, self-centeredness, deficient ego strength and intense narcissistic needs in general as predominating in the "falling in love" process, with such individuals being prone to choose partners with complementary needs and/or relatively equivalent levels of emotional maturity, and to over-idealize these partners. (That certainly sounds like transference too. . .)

Rand (1957), however, saw romantic love from a slightly different perspective, one wherein the lover views the beloved as a reflection and personification of the lover's highest values, ideals, and standards. (Upon closer inspection, even that seems like it might be a form of transference. . . .) Yet Kernberg (1978) indicated that the capability to idealize—and re-idealize—another is also a vital indicator of mental health, and that the incapacity to do so is indicative of severe psychopathology.

Romantic (transference) love must, of course, be differentiated from mature, realistic love. In the latter, there is a valuing, a selfless valuing, of the other as a unique, fallible, separate human being in his or her own right, a person with separate and different needs, values, and rights. The capability to love another in this manner is seen as being roughly proportionate to the extent of one's emotional maturity (Fromm, 1956; Fromme, 1965; Peele, 1975; Meissner, 1978; Buscaglia, 1972). In actuality, I would expect one's view of one's beloved is most often some combination or blend of romantic love and realistic love, which is certainly in keeping with Kernberg's (1978) views and with the concept that emotional maturity exists along a continuum of intensity rather than as a black-or-white entity.

Indeed Fromme (1965) indicated that what begins as romantic love often matures to incorporate increasing amounts of realistic love, with romantic love serving the very useful function of bridging the fearsome gap between self-love and other-love.

As I said before, I am a fallible and vulnerable human being. I am not Wonder Woman. I doubt that all my early narcissistic needs were ever fully met. I am aware of the underlying dynamics of romantic love. I have also, over the years, acquired vast amounts of self-awareness. I know that I fall in love from time to time—not very often, but it happens.

I also know that I am not a person given to casual encounters of any kind. I am either committed to a relationship or I can't be bothered, and I cannot feel personally committed to another unless I feel I know that person well and I am in love with that person. As irrational a criterion as that may be, that's where it's at. To choose by any other method would be to make a cold, rational, impersonal, calculating choice, to say, in essence, "I'll start a relationship with *that* one, because it will be good for me," Like spinach. Like vitamin pills.

I realize that the probabilities are stacked against my ever falling in love with a client, not only from the standpoint of my own dynamics (it's a rather rare occurrence in my life under any circumstances) but from the fact that—well, it's just unlikely.

But it could happen. And then I wonder what I would do. It is immediately apparent to me that the professional relationship would have to be terminated; that I could no longer provide the objectivity necessary to properly assist this client. I also believe my client would deserve honesty from me, and would get it. A referral might be in order, if appropriate. My client's overall needs and well-being would certainly have to supersede my own. All this is in keeping with the guidelines proposed by Van Hoose and Kottler (1977) in their discussion of ethics for the mental health practitioner.

I suppose, beyond that, the decision about whether or not to initiate a personal relationship would have to rest on various situational factors. First of all, I realize that the burden of responsibility would be upon me, as the professional, to exercise judgment and restraint, to not do anything to jeopardize the emotional well-being of my client. I also know, in dealing with issues laden with emotion, rationality has a tendency to fly right out the window, making it all the more difficult to realistically assess and deal with such a situation. First, there would have to be a decision as to whether or not the pursuit of a personal relationship would be in my client's best interests and, secondly, in my own best interests. The tendency for clients to idealize their therapists has certainly been well documented (Van Hoose & Kottler, 1977; Black, 1976; Brammer & Shostrom, 1977; Goldman & Milman, 1978), and so there would be my own fear that this person was seeing me as some exaggerated ideal of perfection and not as I really am, i.e., via total transference. Therefore, I suppose I would have to explore this area, to check out that client's reality testing of me, to sort out the proportions of realistic perceptions and transference perceptions. I would also have to sift through and categorize my own needs and perceptions. And then choose and act accordingly.

I also think, were I to decide I sincerely wanted to pursue a relationship, I would be inclined to postpone further contact with that person for several months, to let emotional intensities lessen, and to ultimately allow both of us to more realistically assess one another and any relationship potential that may then exist. That would certainly allow reality factors of various kinds to intercede and perhaps be the most viable alternative. I would certainly never want to enter any relationship based on false premises and perceptions—my own or another's, and could never allow myself to capitalize on another person's vulnerabilities (namely, dependencies, projections, idealizations, etc.). That's just not my personal style.

Most of all, I sincerely hope this dilemma is one that I never have to face!

REFERENCE

Blanck, G. Psychoanalytic technique. In B. Wolman (Ed.), *The Therapist's Handbook: Treatment Methods of Mental Disorders*. NY: Van Nostrand Reinhold Company, 1976.

Brammer, L., & Shostrom, E. *Therapeutic Psychology: Fundamentals of Counseling and Psychotherapy, 3rd Edition.* Englewood Cliffs NJ: Prentice-Hall, Inc.

Fromm, E. *The Art of Loving.* NY: Bantam Books, 1956.

Fromme, A. *The Ability to Love.* North Hollywood CA: Wilshire Book Company, 1965.

Goldman, G. & Milman, D. *Psychoanalytic Psychotherapy.* Reading MA: Addison-Wesley Publishing Company, 1978.

Hendrick, I. *Facts and Theories of Psychoanalysis.* NY: Dell Publishing Company, 1958.

Kernberg, O. Why some people can't love. *Psychology Today, 12*(1), 54–59.

May, R. *Love and Will.* NY: Dell Publishing Company, 1969.

Meisser, W. The conceptualization of marriage and family dynamics from a psychoanalytic perspective. In T. Paolino, Jr. & B. McCrady (Eds.), *Marriage and Marital Therapy.* NY: Brunner/Mazel, Publishers, 1978.

Peele, S. *Love and Addiction.* NY: Signet New American Library, 1975.

Polster, E. & Poster, M. *Gestalt Therapy Integrated.* NY: Vintage Books, 1974.

Rand, A. *Atlas Shrugged.* NY: Signet New American Library, 1957.

Reik, T. *The Need to be Loved.* NY: Bantam Books, 1963.

Tarachow, S. *An Introduction to Psychotherapy.* NY: International Universities Press, Inc., 1963.

Van Hoose, W. & Kottler, W. *Ethical and Legal Issues in Counseling and Psychotherapy.* San Francisco: Jossey-Bass, Publishers, 1977.

Pretrial Diversion: Ethical Issues For The Mental Health Practitioner

CHAPTER 9

CHARLES J. O'LEARY

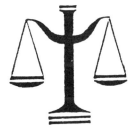

PRETRIAL DIVERSION: ETHICAL ISSUES FOR THE MENTAL HEALTH PRACTITIONER

9

Charles J. O'Leary

Pretrial diversion refers to programs legislated to give first offenders and persons arrested for victimless crimes, such as the possession of marijuana, the choice of accepting a referral to a community therapeutic or educational program rather than facing trial and possible sentencing within the court system.

Typically, acceptance of diversion involves waiving of the right to trial, completion of the community program, and avoidance of any future conviction for a period of six months to two years. In return, the individual is not prosecuted, is not on probation, and eventually has all records of the offense expunged. In California, according to the Penal Code, Section 1001.5, the offense "is deemed never to have occurred."

Most diversion statutes have clear-cut eligibility requirements for participation in such programs, although in practice many offenders are sent to diversion as a result of pretrial bargaining which involves the reduction of charges to fit the requirements (Lampkin, 1980).

Community programs vary greatly, ranging from minimum impact treatment such as attendance at drug diversion classes, to full-scale employment readiness programs (*Yale Law Journal*, 1974). An example of a typical program is one which involves therapeutic intake and the assignment of an offender to a series of self-help and educational groups or to individual counseling, depending on the needs of the individual (Weiss & Sargent, 1976).

Legal and Ethical Issues

A survey of articles on diversion in the legal and criminal justice literature reveals that concern centers around two major issues: (1) the effectiveness of diversion in reaching the stated goals (Rausch, 1978), and (2) the potential for violation of the civil rights of participants in these programs (*Yale Law Journal*, 1974).

Both critics and proponents of diversion speak of the overwhelmingly positive response to the diversion concept. It has been called a "noble experiment" (Schulman, 1973, p. 80), and the rapidity of its implementation and extent of its use are almost universally cited (Rausch, 1978). Among its expected outcomes are: the clearing of court dockets to allow time and expense to be devoted to more serious crimes; the opportunity to reduce recidivism by constructive rehabilitation of potential offenders detected early; and a productive partnership between the criminal justice system and the community.

Proponents of the program claim that those outcomes are in fact being met. They have compared recidivism rates of offenders granted diversion with those individuals processed through the courts before diversion was implemented. Those individuals granted diversion did better (Department of Justice, State of California, 1978). Proponents also point to program reports on therapeutic change for participants through education and treatment (Weiss & Sargent, 1976). These reports mention favorable outcomes, such as early detection and screening of persons with psychosocial problems who would otherwise go untreated. It has been argued that the overall outcome of diversion is vastly superior for the individual simply because "it frees the defendant from pretrial detention and allows him the freedom of living and moving in the community" (Skoler, 1974, p. 485).

Critics of such programs, however, seem more numerous in the legal literature. Their primary objection is the lack of solid research done on outcomes, especially in view of the phenomenal increase in the number of such programs. Rausch (1978, p. 80) pointed out that the "of course it works" attitude on the part of the community and treatment personnel blocks objective research on "what treatment, by whom, is most effective for this individual with that specific problem and under what set of circumstances."

Rausch and other writers (*Yale Law Journal,* 1974) argue that effectiveness can only be measured through the creating of "control groups either sent through the criminal justice system or diverted without treatment" (Rausch, 1978, p. 76). Resistance to this type of research is strong, both for financial and manpower reasons and for ethical reasons. For example, it would be unfair to discriminate against individuals merely for the sake of research (Weiss & Sargent, 1976). Other authors point out that some programs meet diversion goals in measurable ways and others do not, and that evaluation must be made specific for each program.

Questions regarding denial of rights of individuals assigned to diversion programs are numerous in the literature. Rather than reducing the number of people prosecuted for minor or victimless crimes, diversion has resulted in widening the nets, thereby pulling into processing and treatment individuals who would otherwise have a low probability of prosecution (McSparo, 1976). The *Yale Law Journal* (1974) discussed three traditional categories of offenders: (1) those who would be automatically screened out of any legal processing; (2) those who have committed offenses which could be prosecuted but are good risks for minimal punitive attention; and (3) those who should be clearly prosecuted. It was cautioned that diversion may be seriously misused if applied to those individuals in the first or third categories.

Duree (1974) argued that diversion statutes give the district attorney the power of judge and jury. In other words, in many cases the district attorney alone decides who is eligible for diversion and who is not, thereby conducting "de facto" trials without a defense. A related concern is the way clients waive their right to trial. The choice of diversion is often presented to defendants in an attractive way immediately after the stress of arrest. Thus there is the possibility that even innocent persons or those arrested without due regard for their rights might be hurried into a program "for their own good" at the cost of constitutional rights.

It may be concluded from this review that the idea of diversion is popular and is an appealing alternative to the "crime" of punishment, but that its effectiveness has not been sufficiently proved by objective research which justifies its widespread implementation. More research by both criminal justice representatives and the participating community programs is strongly indicated. Questions of individual participants' civil rights should be continually raised, both at the level of the court system and by practitioners working within the community programs.

Responsibilities of the Mental Health Practitioner

Although the state, represented by the court system, has the responsibility for the legality and appropriateness of its referrals, mental health practitioners are responsible for their acceptance of that referral and must function within the ethical standards of the profession. Two issues of ethical practice are relevant here: responsibility, and client welfare.

Psychologists "accept responsibility for the consequences of their work and make every effort to insure that their services are used appropriately" (American Psychological Association, 1979). The practitioner must be aware that the courts can deal only with persons according to external norms and are not competent generally to refer according to individual needs or particular problems. Therefore, the practitioner must provide treatment that is appropriate to the individual. An intake procedure is of great importance to insure that the treatment procedure will fit the individual needs of the client (Weiss & Sargent, 1976).

All treatment procedures must be flexible enough to meet the varied needs of individuals who have limited or serious personal problems. Practitioners must neither treat someone if the problems are beyond their competence, nor apply treatment procedures where there are no problems. Legal labels can never be considered therapeutic. One example of unethical conduct would be to place a person arrested for marijuana usage in a treatment program for drug addicts.

"Psychologists respect the integrity and protect the welfare of the people and groups with whom they work. When there is a conflict of interest between the client and the psychologist's employing institution, psychologists clarify the nature and direction of their loyalties and responsibilities and keep all parties informed of their commitments" (American Psychological Association, 1979).

Mental health practitioners must be agents for the individual client. In diversion programs, they are also agents for the state in that they are usually given power to determine and report on the client's compliance with the agreed-upon conditions for diversion. In fulfillment of this dual role, again the intake seems of prime importance and should include the establishment of a contract (Corey, Corey, & Callanan, 1979). The client must be informed of the court's expectations of the practitioner, especially where they might conflict with the client's interests, such as the programs's inability to keep information confidential. A treatment plan must be formulated which meets both the court's requirements and the individual's needs. The individual must have every right to turn down the plan and return to court.

It would be unethical for the practitioner to create a treatment plan which exceeds the client's needs; to create a climate in which refusal of the plan was made difficult, especially by vague communication; to accept for treatment individuals who are innocent of the original charges and are unaware of their rights in the matter; or to misuse one's professional authority by any explicit or implicit diagnoses not specifically contracted for by the client. To state these principles more positively, it is the ethical obligation of therapists to relate to the divertee as they would to any client; that is, they place at the client's disposal their therapeutic skills in such a way that the client has maximum freedom and is treated with maximum respect.

Gray Areas of Practitioner's Participation in Diversion

Although a state of clarity may be reached on certain ethical issues, mental health practitioners involved in pretrial diversion are sometimes faced with problems which are difficult to resolve. They are in the position of serving two masters, and, secondly, they are often confronted with people involved in minor, victimless crimes in which any involvement of the state is questionable.

A third problem is that diversion represents both a welcome involvement of helping persons in the criminal justice system and a potential step in the direction of Szasz's "therapeutic state." Finally, the therapist is participating in an endeavor whose effectiveness is essentially unproven at this point in time. The resolution of such issues is only possible in terms of individual ethical behavior, particularly with regard to clear communication with all parties involved. Such a resolution may bring peace of soul but does not solve the problem.

Treatment programs that focus, as most seem to do, on individual goals for clients rather than any state-imposed goals seem most congruent with therapeutic ethics. How then are these programs serving the society which funds them? A program which deals with marijuana users who continue to be marijuana users, but do not get arrested again and may even improve in other areas of functioning, may be considered effective in one sense, even though it fails in its implicit outcome. Would it be better for professionals to refuse to accept such an implied outcome (instead of seeking more reasonable de facto outcomes) and thus throw back to society the need for further public discussion and changed legislation?

The problem of the creation of a therapeutic state is appropriately raised whenever something is legislated "for one's own good." Would it be better, or at least more respectful of an individual's rights, to punish deviant behavior or to ignore it, but never to use it to involve the state in mandating an individual's treatment or self-improvement? Again, would therapists' refusal to have anything to do with mandated treatment bring about needed discussion of societal norms and individual's rights?

Conclusions

The writer has worked in diversion programs, both for adults and juveniles, for seven years. Participation in these programs involves a thorough intake for the client who is then assigned to one of two programs: a series of four to six week educational sessions, or individual counseling. Determination of program is made on the basis of need and motivation for treatment.

The educational sessions have evolved over the years and have been greatly influenced by participants' written and verbal critiques. A series of self-help classes and structured groups directed at the development needs of the participants have been added to the drug and legal education facets. Since the modal participant is in his or her early twenties, the focus in these groups is on identity, vocational matters, and intimacy concerns. Great care is taken to invite involvement and respect, as well as to assure privacy and personal freedom. Group members frequently refer themselves for further individual or relationship counseling at the end of the initial sessions.

Those assigned to individual counseling develop a contract with the therapist that is similar to contracts drawn up in voluntary therapy sessions. The length, content, and number of sessions are determined by the counselor's ability and the client's need and motivation. Family therapy, relationship therapy, vocational counseling, and long-term group therapy are also available and may be chosen by the client.

Limited research on the program has indicated low recidivism rates among the participants (Department of Justice, State of California, 1978), as well as some gains in other areas of functioning (Weiss & Sargent, 1976).

Subjectively, the program seems right. Clients are treated with respect and freedom. Many opportunities for effective crisis intervention have arisen. Most importantly, the program provides a meaningful personal and educational contact for a population in need of both questioning and support. There is no objective research which supports these observations. In practice, a client's arrest and/or drug use, more often than not indicates a need for therapeutic contact.

Subjectively, the process that leads to the program seems flawed. It is a well-motivated, sensible but highly imperfect response to laws that are the result of a malnourished public dialogue. It is a questionable means to an end that is only made worthwhile through effortful interaction with individuals. Although it is a step in the right direction—that is, toward more effective response to lawbreaking—it is not very steady and has not gone very far.

After considering the issues discussed in this paper, the writer reached a number of personal decisions: (1) to continue to work in diversion programs; (2) to pay more attention to *the clients' understanding of the legal process and their rights within it;* (3) to increase communication with authorities in charge of diversion programs, supporting current attempts at better research; and (4) to encourage officials to use diversion for populations with whom it may be more needed and effective, for example child abusers, repeating offenders, and property offenders.

REFERENCES

Agopian, R. Evaluation of adult diversion programs: The California experience. *Federal Probation*, 1977, *41*, 15–18.

American Psychological Association. *Ethical Standards of Psychologists*, Washington DC: Author, 1979.

Bahnsted, M. Answers to three questions about juvenile diversion. *Journal of Research in Criminology,* 1978, *15*(1), 109–123.

Corey, G., Corey, M., & Callanan, P. *Professional and Ethical Issues in Counseling and Psychotherapy*, Monterey: Brooks/Cole, 1979.

Cohen, S. Marijuana: A new ball game? *Drug Abuse and Alcoholism Newsletter*, 1979, *8*(4).

Department of Justice, State of California. *Drug diversion recidivism*. Sacramento CA: Bureau of Criminal Statistics, February, 1978.

Duree, J. Diversion and the judicial function, *Pacific Law Journal*, July 1974, *5*(2), 764–784.

Lampkin, A. Personal Communication, Research Coordinator, Department of Drug Programs, County of San Diego, 1980.

McSparro, J. Community correction and diversion, *Crime and Delinquency*, 1976, *26*(2), 226–247.

Roesch, R. Does adult diversion work? Failure of research in criminal justice, *Crime and Delinquency*, 1978, *24*(1), 72–80.

Salmon, R. An analysis of public marijuana policy, *Social Casework*, 1972, *1*, 53–60.

Schulman, M. Diversion— A noble experiment, *Orange County Bar Journal*, 1973, *1*, 80–91.

Skoler, D. Protecting the rights of defendants in pretrial intervention programs, *Criminal Law Bulletin*, 1974, *10*(6), 473–492.

Van Hoose, W. & Kottler, J. *Ethical and legal issues in counseling and psychotherapy*. San Francisco: Jossey/Bass, 1977.

Weiss, A. & Sargent, G. *Mental health and criminal justice diversion: partnership for community change*. Washington DC: American Psychological Association convention, 1976.

Yale Law Journal, Pretrial diversion from the criminal process, author, 1974, *83*(4), 827–854.

Confidentiality In
Group Therapy

CHAPTER 10

JAN MELLINGER

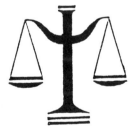

CONFIDENTIALITY IN GROUP THERAPY

10

Jan Mellinger

When persons decide to enter psychotherapy, they may choose group counseling. They may make their decision on the basis of economics, type of therapy offered, or availability of a specific therapist. While these criteria might make group counseling the therapy of choice, the person must consider the issue of confidentiality as it relates to group counseling. Will the information the person divulges be privileged in either a social, moral, or legal sense? What are the rights of a group member regarding confidentiality? These issues arouse a great deal of legal and ethical controversy and are only beginning to be resolved.

California state law recognizes the psychotherapist-patient privilege.

> . . . the patient, whether or not a party, has a privilege to refuse to disclose, and to prevent another from disclosing, a confidential communication between patient and psychotherapist if the privilege is claimed by: (a) the holder of the privilege; (b) a person who is authorized to claim the privilege by the holder of the privilege; or (c) the person who was the psychotherapist at the time of the confidential communication (California Evidence Code, Section 1014 et seq.).

State law also recognizes privilege for confidential marital communications which states, in part:

> . . . a spouse . . . has a privilege during the marital relationship and afterwards to refuse to disclose, and to prevent another from disclosing, a communication if he claims the

privilege and the communication was made in confidence between him and the other spouse while they were husband and wife (California Evidence Code, Section 980).

There are some exceptions to this rule. When the therapist is counseling a husband and wife, confidentiality applies to this "small group" relationship. The husband and wife are protected from each other's disclosures and disclosures made by the psychotherapist. However, when a husband and wife choose to go into group therapy, the marital privilege no longer applies. The law may be deemed to mean that the privilege may be asserted to prevent testimony by anyone, including eavesdroppers. Precedents show that this is not the case in practice. In *People v. Peak* (1944), the decision states, in part:

> The purpose of Section 1881 of the Code Civil Procedure (now Evidence Code, Section 980) is to hold intact the confidence which naturally arises from the relationship of husband and wife. It is not the act of communication but the substance thereof that is held legally inviolate. . . a third person who overhears a communication between a husband and wife, whether with or without their knowledge, and whether surreptitiously or openly, may testify regarding what he thus learned, although the communication may be, as between the husband and wife, one of a confidential character. (Id. at p. 903, 904).

This seeming violation of confidentiality is covered by the provisions on waiver by disclosure which states:

> . . . the right of any person to claim a privilege provided by Section. . . 980 (privilege for confidential marital communications), . . . 1014 (psychotherapist–patient privilege), . . . is waived with respect to a communication protected by such privilege if any holder of the privilege, without coercion, has disclosed a significant part of the communication or has consented to such disclosure made by anyone (California Evidence Code, Section 912).

In group therapy, then, what we are left with is no protection under the law for confidentiality. The question arises whether confidentiality is important in the group therapy setting. Meyer and Smith (1977) conducted a study of university students in which the students were asked their opinions of group confidentiality. The questions were designed as follows:

Presume that you have now decided to seek entry into a different therapy group and this therapist tells you that information discussed in the group would *not* be considered confidential. Would you:

(a) Decide not to enter group therapy?
(b) Enter the group, but with substantially less inclination to reveal relevant information in the group?
(c) Enter the group with approximately the same motivation and feelings you had before the therapist's statements?
(d) Enter the group with even greater motivation and willingness to reveal relevant information (Meyer & Smith, 1977, p. 32)?

The students were asked the same question except told that the group members were pledged to confidentiality. To the question of no confidentiality, 81.8% answered "a" or "b." When confidentiality was pledged, 47.2% answered "a" or "b." The conclusion which Meyer and Smith (1977, p. 32) drew, states:

> ... that based on the expectancies of these respondents, either statement on confidentiality would be likely to lessen the effectiveness of the group therapy process because of both an inclination to avoid entering therapy and a loss of substantial information to the group. When the therapist states that "confidentiality" does not exist, there is rather an extreme loss.

This does not mean the issue of confidentiality is one to be shuffled to the background. Rather, therapists must realistically examine what options would best serve the interest of the group and realize the possible legal ramifications of their decision.

Several attempts have been made to legally clarify the group confidentiality question. California state law regarding confidential communication between patient and psychotherapist states, in part:

> ... information... transmitted between a patient and his psychotherapist in the course of that relationship and in confidence by a means which, so far as the patient is aware, discloses the information to no third persons other than those who are present to further the interest of the patient in the consultation or examination (California Evidence Code, Section 1012).

It must be determined if members of a group can be considered to be aiding in the diagnosis and treatment of the person claiming the privilege. Rule 504 of the Federal Rules of Evidence addresses itself more directly to the problem:

> A patient has a privilege to refuse to disclose and to prevent another person from disclosing confidential communications made for the purposes of diagnosis or treatment of his mental or emotional condition, including drug addiction, among himself, his psychotherapist, or persons who are participating in the diagnosis or treatment under direction of the psychotherapist, including members of the patient's family.

Both these laws are ambiguous at best and leave interpretation to the discretion of the court. One case which sheds some light on the problem is *Grosslight v. Superior Court*. The decision stated, in part:

> The psychotherapist-patient privilege under Evidence Code 1014, is to be liberally construed in favor of the patient. The psychotherapist-patient privilege (Evidence Code 1014) covers all relevant communications by the patient's intimate family members to psychotherapists and to psychiatric personnel, including secretaries who take histories for the purpose of recording statements for the use of psychiatrists.

Although still not extending privilege to a group, *Grosslight* extends the privilege beyond just the therapist and the client. In doing so, it expands the limitations of privilege and conceivably opens the door for further expansion.

All that has been discussed so far seems to leave our poor patient in limbo. Patients merely want the assurance that their innermost thoughts will not become headline news. It would appear that under current law, the therapist cannot guarantee this will not happen. Since group therapy is a popular form of psychotherapy, we need to explore some of the options in maintaining group confidentiality.

It would be ideal if a simple explanation of confidentiality to the group would suffice. Certainly Client A does not want his or her revelations exposed and therefore should be aware that Client B should be awarded the same respect. Yet, it is not human nature to be quite so altruistic, especially considering some of the good "cocktail party" material picked up in groups.

The method that appears to be gaining popularity is having a contractual agreement among all members of the group. Violation of this contract could result in a civil suit (tort or breach of contract) against individual members of the group.

In a recent decision, the legality of the group contract was upheld. A woman, Gwen Davis, enrolled herself in a nude therapy group under the guise of being a client. She signed the group contract. Later, she published a thinly disguised "novel" of the group experience, called *Touching*. The therapist, Dr. Paul Bindrim, was accused by other professionals of allowing the expose and thereby setting his patients up for public ridicule. Bindrim, with full knowledge of his patients, had tape recorded the sessions. When the matter went to court, these tape recordings would be the solid evidence which decided the case. Bindrim sued Davis for fraud, breach of contract, and libel. Fraud could not be proven to the satisfaction of the jury. Breach of contract was awarded by the superior court but disallowed by the appellate court, which reasoned that the patient had the right to report on the treatment she had received. It should be noted that this limitation would not have applied, had the suit been brought by another group member. The libel suit brought an award for $75,000 in punitive damages.

The tape recordings that Dr. Bindrim had made during the session established that Ms Davis had written, in effect, a report of the session. The names of the participants had been changed, but much of the text was matched in content to the tape.

Dr. Bindrim (180, p. 2) stated:

> ... I believe that therapists can significantly reduce the risk of unauthorized disclosure of confidential material by first, requiring that all participants sign a confidentiality agreement, and second, by making recordings of the sessions in full view of all participants and keeping the tapes on file.

The therapist must have a contract that is both understandable and legal. An attorney could clarify the necessary items to be included and assure contract legality. Morrison, Federico, and Rosenthal (1975, p. 7) proposed the following contract for practitioners in the state of California:

> We, the undersigned, in consideration of and in return for receiving group psychotherapy and its possible benefits, and in consideration and return for similar promises by

other members of the psychotherapy group, consciously and willingly promise never to reveal the identity of any group member (listed below) to anyone who is not in (the group), other than the staff of the psychiatric agency from which we receive services. We realize that to relate specific problems of a group member to a non-group member, even though the name of the group member may not be directly revealed, may at times lead to the eventual disclosure of the group member's identity. Therefore, we promise to avoid speaking of any group member's problems in any manner which would even remotely risk revealing the identity of that group member. We fully realize and strongly agree that in the event of a lawsuit for breach of contract, we give the offended party the right to recover for damage to his/her reputation for the minimum amount of $_____. Also, such party may recover for any other damages which can be proven.

Although contractual agreements seem to be the method of choice at this point in time, they do not seem to be the ultimate answer to the problem. The process of having a contract, having the group members sign, and having the option of a civil suit seems to involve the members in the responsibility of confidentiality. However, it is a rather roundabout method of insuring confidentiality in groups. Instead of being directly responsible for violation of confidentiality, the group members are responsible for the terms of a contract. This puts much weight to bear on the contract itself and assurance of its legality is critical.

It appears that a statute which addresses itself directly to the confidentiality in group therapy issue is needed. It is an idea which has been broadening for quite some time. In *Mullen v. United States* (1958, p. 281), the judge stated:

I think a communication made in reasonable confidence that it will not be disclosed, and in such circumstances that disclosure is shocking to the moral sense of the community, should not be disclosed in a judicial proceeding, whether the trusted person is or is not a wife, husband, doctor, lawyer, or minister.

Geiser and Rheingold (1964, p. 831) suggested the following provision:

A client, or his authorized representative, has a privilege to prevent a witness from disclosing in any judicial, administrative, or legislative proceeding, communications pertaining to the diagnosis or treatment of the client's mental or emotional disorder, or difficulty in personal or social adjustment, between the client and any of the following: a member of the mental health profession, any other professional or lay person who participates with such a member of a mental health profession in the accomplishment of individual or group diagnosis or treatment, or members of the client's family, or between any of these persons as concerns diagnosis or treatment.

Until a statute similar to the aforementioned provision is adopted, the status of confidentiality in group therapy remains in limbo. In California, an individual is protected by psychotherapist-patient privilege. Married couples are protected under their own confidentiality statute. Individuals in group therapy at this time must rely on roundabout methods to insure confidentiality.

What is clearly needed is new legislation which defines privilege in relation to group therapy. This legislation is needed both on the state and national level. In order for group therapy to be maintained as an effective form of treatment, the client must have a guarantee of confidentiality. Legal protection of that right is the desirable conclusion.

REFERENCES

Bindrim, P. Group therapy: Protecting privacy, *Psychology Today, 14*(2), July 1980.

Foster, L. Group psychotherapy: A pool of legal witnesses? *International Journal of Group Psychotherapy*, 1975 *XXV*(1), 50.

Geiser, R. & Rheingold, P. Psychology and the legal process: Testimonial privileged communication, *American Psychologist, 19*, 1964, 831–837.

Grosslight v. Superior Court of Los Angeles County, 72 C.A.3d 502, 140 Cal. Rptr 278 (1977).

Myer, R. & Smith, S. A crisis in group therapy, *American Psychologist, 32,* 1977, 32.

Morrison, J., Federico, M., & Rosenthal, H. Contracting confidentiality in group psychotherapy, *Journal of Forensic Psychology, 7,* 1975.

Mullen v. United States, 263 F.2d 275, (1958).

People v. Peak, 153 P.2d 464, 66 C.A.2d 894, 1944.

Schwitzgebel, R. & Schwitzgebel, R. *Law and Psychological Practice*, NY: John Wiley & Sons, 1980.

Token Economies In Institutional Settings

CHAPTER 11

JOHN M. HENNING

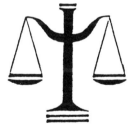

TOKEN ECONOMIES IN INSTITUTIONAL SETTINGS

11

John M. Henning

Token economies are a widely used form of behavioral treatment in institutional and educational settings. In recent years, however, the courts have placed restrictions on the uses of token economies and on what kind of behaviors can be manipulated in a token economy. This chapter focuses on the theory behind the workings of token economies as well as their practical applications. Also, court decisions regarding token economies are presented and the implications of these decisions discussed.

Schwitzgebel and Schwitzgebel defined a token economy as "an environmental arrangement, normally found in institutional settings, whereby tokens and similar evidence of earned credits are used to purchase items, services, and privileges" (Schwitzgebel & Schwitzgebel, 1980, p. 111).

Token economies are based on the behavioral laws of operant conditioning which were formalized in the works of B.F. Skinner. The primary law of operant conditioning is that behavior is strengthened or weakened by its consequences (Wexler, 1973). A client's behavior is changed by reinforcing certain target behaviors. In this way, the client's behavior is "shaped." This shaping takes place through the use of secondary reinforcers or generalized reinforcers. That is, when clients engage in one of the target behaviors, they are given a secondary reinforcer, usually tokens or points. These secondary reinforcers can then be converted into primary reinforcers, such as snacks, clothes, or privileges. In this way, the primary reinforcers strengthen the target behaviors.

The selection of appropriate primary reinforcers has at times been a problem. If clients are not interested in the snacks or privileges offered to them, they will not engage in the target behaviors. This motivational problem is explained by the Premack Principle, which states that "if one activity occurs more frequently than another, it will be an effective reinforcer for that other activity" (Whaley & Malott, 1971, p. 316). If a child spends more time watching television than reading, for example, then according to this principle, watching television will be an effective reinforcer for reading.

The use of token economies has been widespread. Prisons and mental hospitals were the first to use token economy systems, followed shortly by institutions for the developmentally disabled and agencies working with delinquents. Today they are used in colleges, public school classrooms, psychological clinics, and agencies dealing with many different populations.

When token economies were first implemented, it was assumed that when rewards rather than punishments were employed, no grave legal, social or ethical questions were involved (Wexler, 1973). In institutions that dealt with chronic mental patients or the developmentally disabled the target behaviors were work assignments and self-care behaviors such as grooming, bathing, toothbrushing, bed-making, etc. Token economies seemed to be a good way to combat the apathy and dependency fostered by institutionalization. In that respect token economies were highly successful, but the problem arose in that one of the target responses of most token economies is adequate functioning on an institutional work assignment. Many persons objected to requiring patients to work for mental institutions (Wexler, 1973). Requiring patients to engage in certain target behaviors in order to obtain meals or a bed also drew criticism.

Many law suits were filed regarding treatment and human rights issues, but the most extensive specification of rights came from *Wyatt v. Stickney* (Wexler, 1973). In that decision the court barred all involuntary patient labor involving hospital operation and maintenance, whether therapeutic or not, but permitted voluntary institutional work of either a therapeutic or nontherapeutic nature so long as the labor was compensated pursuant to the federal minimum wage law.

Additionally, the *Wyatt v. Stickney* decision made certain rights that had been previously viewed as contingent rights to be earned in a token economy into absolute rights that were basic to institutionalized patients. These included the following:

- Visit and make phone calls
- Send sealed mail
- Wear own clothes
- Attend religious services
- Interact with the opposite sex
- Take a shower and use the toilet in privacy
- Use day room area with reading lamps, television, and other recreational facilities
- Have a comfortable bed, a closet or locker, a chair, and a bedside table
- Have frequent changes of bedding and other linen
- Have meals in dining room
- Have an individualized treatment plan
- Have appropriate treatment for mental disorders and physical illness
- Have transitional treatment and care when released from the hospital
- Have a humane psychological and physical environment that is comfortable and safe (Schwitzgebel, 1980, p. 113)
- Have the right to exercise physically several times weekly and to be outdoors regularly and frequently
- Have a right to the least restrictive conditions necessary to achieve the purposes of commitment (Wexler, 1973, p. 94)

In that decision the court specifically informed mental health and behavior modification practitioners what rights were not to be used as contingencies in token economies. This restriction might have put a damper on many institutional treatment programs were it not for the strong statements regarding right to treatment.

The purpose of involuntary hospitalization for treatment purposes is treatment and not mere custodial care or punishment. This is the only justification from a constitutional standpoint that allows civil commitments to mental institutions (Singletary et al., 1977, p. 136).

This same opinion was echoed by the court in the case of *Ragsdale v. Overhalser*, which stated:

> Adequate and effective treatment is constitutionally required because, absent treatment, the hospital is transformed into a penitentiary where one could be held indefinitely for no convicted offense (Singletary, 1977, p. 136).

These decisions placed a heavy burden on institutional staff. They were told they had to provide treatment to patients. Moreover, the treatment could not be the same as the methods they had been using. Many behavioral psychologists had problems understanding the expansion and protection of patient rights. One reason for this lack of understanding was that the law relies on concepts of freedom and dignity, but these concepts are meaningless to behavioral psychologists in the mold of B. F. Skinner. The law speaks to our right to privacy without which we may lose our very integrity as persons. We must be allowed to respect, love, trust, feel affection for others, and not regard ourselves as objects (Di Giacomo, 1977). The court decisions refer to human dignity. Man should be "as Nature or God intended him to be and is therefore inviolable" (Di Giacomo, 1977, p. 104).

Token economies threaten human dignity, freedom and privacy. Behavioral psychologists point out that infants are under the social control of their parents and are heavily socialized in the ways of their particular culture or subculture.

If freedom and dignity can be equated with freedom to choose one's own behavior, then Ayllan, a behavior psychologist, offers some insight into token economies, patient rights, and freedom.

> The aspect of choice in the token economy is of crucial importance. Choice, to be meaningful, must allow the person to achieve the consequences attendant upon choosing one thing over another. When the individual discovers that his desires will be respected he will learn that he must bear the consequences of his own choice and he will, in turn, learn responsibility for his own actions (Ayllan, 1975, p. 15).

After the consequences of alternative choices have been outlined to the client, then it is crucial that his or her choice be respected. Only in this way can the demeaning and eroding of the client's self-respect and dignity be avoided and the responsibility for his or her own actions be assumed.

This explanation seems to resolve some of the theoretical problems involved in the court decisions, but there remain pragmatic considerations concerning *Wyatt v. Stickney* that are unresolved. There is a dilemma regarding chronic mental patients and low functioning developmentally disabled clients. These people respond only to the most primitive reinforcers; that is, food, but food is protected under *Wyatt v. Stickney* (Wexler, 1973). As an answer to this, Friedman (1975) suggested that under appropriate circumstances the basic rights of *Wyatt v. Stickney* are waivable just as any basic right is waivable. Where legitimate *parens patriae* justification exists, it may be appropriate for the state to waive certain basic rights on behalf of incompetent patients. In cases where the state does not have this justification, the waiving of rights would be the responsibility of the guardian. Another problem deals with patients who know they can attain the necessities and some of the luxuries of life for free. Then it becomes difficult to motivate them to participate in a treatment program or to encourage them to leave the institution.

It has been suggested that the courts are looking at two questions regarding treatment programs: (1) how aversive is the treatment program, and (2) how effective is this treatment? (Greenberg & Meagher, 1977).

If the treatment program is the most effective treatment available, it may be allowed to continue even if it is somewhat more aversive than other treatment programs that are not as effective. For this reason research comparing token economy treatment and other forms of treatment is very important. Research comparing the feelings of patients about different types of treatment is also important.

Another problem centers around the working of patients in institutions. There is evidence that establishing work as a target behavior is therapeutic rather than merely cost-saving to the institution (Wexler, 1973). That is, work is therapeutic in preventing boredom and institutionalization. It has been suggested that periodic job rotation would help prevent abuse of labor for institutional maintenance. Also, no patient should be allowed to obtain a position for which he or she alone was qualified (Wexler, 1973).

Ayllan has suggested guidelines for patient participation in token economies that protect the rights of the patient:

- The patient should be informed of the possible outcome of the treatment. A written contract is best.

- The patient should be informed of the procedure that will be used in the treatment.
- The patient should be made to feel that he or she is free to choose whether or not to participate in the program.
- The patient should be able at any time to discontinue his or her participation in the program without incurring prejudice or penalty.
- Information necessary to make a decision to discontinue treatment should be given to the patient. That is, timely progress reports should be given to the patient.
- The patient is entitled to treatment which is suited to his or her individual needs.
- The patient should be given the opportunity to express his or her feelings, views, and attitudes towards the program.
- Only behavioral techniques that enrich the patient's environment beyond a base guarantee of certain social and personal rights should be employed (Ayllan, 1975, p. 11).

In summary, then, this chapter examined token economies as they apply in institutional settings specifically. Initially their theoretical underpinnings were explained. Next, the findings in the *Wyatt v. Stickney* case were presented along with problems and solutions regarding patient rights and token economies. The courts have answered many questions about human rights and treatment, but many questions remain unanswered.

Will patients be able to waive some of their rights? Will the state be able to waive some rights for the patients? What will happen to chronic longterm patients who refuse conventional treatment or who do not respond to conventional treatment? Do the same standards of patient rights in institutional settings apply to classrooms as apply to community agencies? Unfortunately, most of these questions still beg answers.

REFERENCES

Akers, R. & Hawkins, R. (Eds.) *Law and Control in Society*. Englewood Cliffs NJ: Prentice-Hall, 1975.

Ayllan, T. Behavior modification in institutional settings, *Arizona Law Review*, 1975, *XVII*, 3–19.

Di Giacoma, R. Behavior modification: Toward the understanding and reform of federal policy, *Corrective and Social Psychiatry and Journal of Behavior Technology: Methods and Therapy,* 1977, *XXIII,* 101–110.

Friedman, P. Legal regulation of applied behavior analysis in mental institutions and prisons, *Arizona Law Review,* 1975, *XVII,* 39–104.

Greenberg, D. & Meagher, R., Jr. The courts and the token economy: An empirical approach to the problem, *Behavior Therapy,* 1977, *viii,* 377–382.

Paul, G. & Lentz, R. *Psychosocial Treatment of Chronic Mental Patients.* Cambridge, Mass: Harvard University Press, 1977.

Schwitzgebel, R. & Schwitzgebel, R. *Law and Psychological Practice.* NY: John Wiley and Sons, 1980.

Singletary, E., Collings, G., & Dennis, H. *Law Briefs on Litigation and the Rights of Exceptional Children, Youth, and Adults.* Washington DC: University Press, 1977.

Tapp, J. & Levine, F. (Eds.) *Law, Justice, and the Individual in Society,* NY: Holt, Rinehart, & Winston, 1977.

Wexler, D. Token and taboo: Behavior modification, token economies, and the law, *California Law Review,* 1973, *LXI,* 81–109.

Whaley, D. & Malott, R. *Elementary Principles of Behavior.* Englewood Cliffs NJ: Prentice-Hall, 1971.

Coercion In Hypnosis: Abuses Of The Client-Hypnotist Relationship

CHAPTER 12

STAN MALKIN

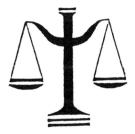

COERCION IN HYPNOSIS: ABUSES OF THE CLIENT-HYPNOTIST RELATIONSHIP

12

Stan Malkin

Hypnosis is a complex process of heightened or aroused concentration. "Although peripheral awareness is reduced in sleep and hypnosis alike, focal awareness, which is rendered almost imperceptible in sleep, is at a maximized capacity in hypnosis" (Friedman, Kaplan & Sadock, 1976, p. 905). Hypnosis has been described as an altered state of intense and sensitive interpersonal relatedness between hypnotist and subject, characterized by the subject's nonrational (but not necessarily irrational) submission and relative abandonment of executive control to a more or less regressed, dissociated state.

In the application of hypnosis to the practice of psychotherapy, the therapist uses the intense, focused awareness of the person to concentrate on certain areas. It is generally agreed that everything done in psychotherapy can be accomplished without hypnosis, but that hypnosis, as a specialized tool, may facilitate and accelerate the impact of the psychotherapeutic intervention (Lichtenstein, 1980).

When therapists commit an error in a nonhypnotic setting, the patients can rely on their own critical faculties to cope with the error to a certain degree. However, this capacity for critical evaluation is not readily available to the patient in the hypnotized state, so that the evaluation and possible correction of the error is postponed or may not be made at all. The existence of such possible conditions make a strong case for the practice of intensive, short-term, insight therapy being undertaken only by well-trained, competent, experienced, and disciplined therapists.

One of the critical questions to consider with regard to ethical principles in the practice of hypnosis is this notion of diminished

165

control. There has been enormous controversy over the issue of diminished control. Questions have been raised regarding whether hypnotists (or any therapists for that matter) have used their prestigious position to unduly influence or coerce patients into performing antisocial or criminal acts, seductions and so on. Research, case studies and discussions in the literature generally concentrate on presenting in great detail, the question of whether there is something inherent to hypnosis and the hypnotic process which reduces the subject's control. If so, is this related to the techniques and processes of hypnosis? Is it related to the question of subject susceptibility, consent and compliance? Or, is there something special or unique about the nature of the relationship between hypnotist and client which leads to various misuses and abuses?

A review and discussion of the literature will clarify these issues as well as shed light on the various ethical considerations which are implicitly involved. I will, therefore, first present a review of the literature regarding this issue of coercion and will follow this with a discussion of the emergent ethical implications.

According to prominent investigators, it is believed that a hypnotized subject cannot be coerced into performing an act which is in violation with his or her values and beliefs (Conn, 1972; Orne, 1972; Wolberg, 1959). A number of equally prestigious authors disagree with this position (Kline, 1972; Watkins, 1972). They contend that antisocial behavior can, in fact, be initiated by hypnosis. It seems that during the time period necessary to discover the difference between the patient's compulsion to comply with the therapist's signal and his or her resistance to it, they may feel confused and unable to exercise their best judgment. During this time patients may commit an act that is somewhat disparate from their usual conduct. Therefore, it is incumbent upon the therapist, under these circumstances, to assume responsibility for the patient. An explosive abreaction may require psychological measures which are restorative in nature.

In the book, *Hypnosis: Is it for You?*, Lewis Wolberg (1972) asserted that there is no danger that hypnosis could be used to initiate antisocial behavior. He held that there are enough safeguards in the normal defenses of subjects to protect them from being exploited by an unscrupulous hypnotist. Wolberg does not pose the question whether *all* subjects have adequate defenses to protect them from manipulation by so-called unscrupulous therapists. In addition, he made anecdotal reference to a story of a physician who, in order to attempt to correct a tipped uterus, conducted a pelvic examination, which he immediately followed by hypnosis for relaxation, and five minutes later "made another attempt to correct the situation" Wolberg, 1972, p. 282). The results were hysterics and a law suit. Amazingly enough, Wolberg's only point was that hysterical patients can make false accusations. He does not say one word in criticism of the physician.

In the eyes of some hypnotists, responsibility for abuses committed under hypnosis seems to rest with the subject. Subjects are often viewed as dependent, compliant, and suggestible. It appears as though it is quite difficult, at times, for practitioners to assume responsibility for their participation in wrongful acts while involved with an individual (Perry, 1979).

John Watkins (1972) maintained that hypnosis evokes both a special state in the client, and a special relationship between client and therapist. He held that if hypnosis is potent enough to initiate constructive behavior, it is also sufficiently powerful to induce the client to move toward antisocial behavior in the hands of an unscrupulous hypnotist. According to Watkins, hypnotic behavior must be considered as being governed by much dynamic interplay between client and therapist, not merely as a special state of consciousness induced by the hypnotist. He referred to other so-called altered states of consciousness such as those evoked by alcohol, psychedelic drugs, and psychomotor epilepsy. He pointed out that crimes have been committed while people have been in these states. Then why should hypnosis, as an altered state phenomenon, be immune to such dangers?

If we examine the relationship side of the question, Wolberg (1972) maintained that it can be demonstrated that people have induced many types of behavior, both social and antisocial in others, through the impact of their personal qualities. The hypnotist or hypnotherapist are usually persons who are most commanding or persuasive in their verbal behavior toward others. Often they are quite successful in eliciting the behaviors desired in their subjects. Why then, Wolberg proposes, is a line drawn which says they cannot induce a given behavior simply because a distinction is made between social and antisocial behavior? Behavior is behavior. He maintains that if the mores of society were so all-encompassing and compelling, there would be little difficulty in enforcing the law, because there would be little crime.

Morris Kleinhauz and his associates (1979) present an interesting case study of psychopathological manifestations which appear to be causally related to the after-effects of stage hypnosis. A middle-aged respected member of a kibbutz who became the subject of an evening's entertainment by a stage hypnotist, suffered a posttraumatic neurosis. The stage hypnotist, unaware of the participant's traumatic childhood during World War II when she and her sister were hidden from the Nazis, requested her to regress to that age. This reactivated a previously successfully repressed trauma and acted as a precipitating factor to the development of a traumatic neurosis which was left untreated and unreferred. The woman was self-referred for adequate psychiatric treatment eleven years later. Despite the abundance of general comments regarding the potential dangers of hypnosis, the authors contended that there are almost no case histories published which document their occurrence and treatment.

Kleinhaus (1979) maintained that the hazards of hypnosis are greatly heightened during stage hypnosis. He stressed that the emphasis is on entertainment rather than on consideration for the protection of the subject's best interests. Another point which should be added is that a subject is placed on stage without any clinical assessment of previous or present history. Seemingly innocent suggestions, such as age regressions, can have significant emotional meaning and can lead to spontaneous, painful and sometimes dangerous abreactions for a subject. Kleinhaus makes a strong case, in my opinion, for the necessity of maintaining professional standards of training, competence and practice for hypnotists.

Milton Kline (1972) explored the role of hypnosis in relation to the production of antisocial behavior. Both specific psychodynamic factors which play a role in creating conditions under which antisocial behavior is possible and the relationship of this kind of behavior to the social context in which it takes place were examined. Particular emphasis was placed on the interaction of two factors: the personality of the therapist and the emergent compliance of the client.

Kline maintained that the personalities of therapists, their commitment to the goal involved without emotional ambivalence, and their confidence in their ability to organize and direct the given behavior, all contribute to the development and maintenance of an intense relationship with the client. Another factor which adds to the intensity of this relationship is the subject's readiness to be easily hypnotized. This is generally called the subject's susceptibility. According to Kline, the relationship between hypnotist and client engenders strong transference of feelings on the part of the client. All of this, he asserts, contributes to a reawakening of a neurotically desired, dependent, compliant and erotically satisfying relationship. In light of the clinical data which he presents, Kline holds that the hypnotic relationship can be a powerful mechanism for eliciting antisocial behavior. The central issue, he claims, appears to be the nature, intensity and the dimension of the hypnotic relationship, rather than to any significant factors which can be attributed to hypnosis per se. In one of the cases Kline presented in which the individual hypnotist in question was a physician who allegedly had sexual relations with his patient, no mention was ever made by the physician of any guilt or concern over the acts in question. Instead, the physician was apparently only concerned with his own welfare.

In 1972, Jacob Conn published a paper addressing the question of the dangers in hypnosis. Based on his vast clinical experience with private psychiatric patients and a review of the opinions of various experts in the field, he concluded that there are no specific dangers associated with hypnosis per se. He maintained that any actual dangers are only those which accompany any psychotherapeutic relationship. In his opinion, hypnosis is not a power or external force which can be used to influence or coerce clients into doing what is suggested by the hypnotist. Rather, it represents a psychological compromise, which is patient-centered, whose goal is to obtain gratification of unacceptable wishes or needs and to avoid condemnation. Specifically, what Conn appears to be saying is that any sexual act, for example, which occurs while the client is under a hypnotic trance is due solely to wish-fulfillment on the part of the subject. It was remarkable to the writer, the lengths to which some researchers go to ignore the fact of complicity on the part of the hypnotist or therapist. I will return to this point later.

Martin Orne maintains there is a

> ... unique quality in the doctor-patient relationship which makes the patient vulnerable and permits the sick and unscrupulous physician to use such a relationship in the service of his own gratification. Hypnosis itself is unlikely to increase the risks to the patient except insofar as it

resonates with the power fantasies of the therapist (Orne, 1972, pp. 112–113).

Orne goes further to suggest the use of a kind of inventory for hypnotists whereby they can check some of their own needs and motives. In the end, he concluded that the patient ultimately retains control, and that hypnosis is a shared enterprise.

By way of concluding this section, I would like to report that I discovered a lengthy and recent report by Campbell Perry (1979) which reviewed the evidence presented in a legal case regarding the issues of coercion and compliance. Specifically, this case involved a lay hypnotist who was found guilty of three sexual offenses against two female clients. Due to the extreme length and complexity of issues involved in this case, I will not attempt to summarize it. Any interested readers are encouraged to read through it on their own. The reason I cite this paper is because it serves to crystallize the various antagonistic viewpoints regarding hypnosis. The author presented segments of verbatim transcripts, not just of the defendant and plaintiff, but of the testimony of expert witnesses.

All expert witnesses involved in this trial as well as the investigators most representative of the different camps, whether they concluded that hypnosis can or cannot be used in a coercive fashion, concurred that hypnosis can be used to activate self-destructive aspects in a disturbed patient. All researchers cited in the paper agreed that abuses which occur in the context of a therapeutic relationship, do so primarily because of the nature of the close interpersonal relationship which is formed. The testimony of the defendant in this particular case was quite consistent with the comments of other defendants, in that he said that if his client were not desirous of his amorous advances, the sexual encounter would never have occurred. This may be technically true, in that it points to the possible compliance of the client in engaging in such acts. However, it completely and remarkably ignores the hypnotist's willingness to go along with such events. In this particular case, the evidence appeared to indicate active and premeditated solicitation of sexual activity through the operation of hypnosis.

It seems apparent that the defendant's behavior violated the ethical principles of the Society for Clinical and Experimental Hypnosis when he clearly fell short of abiding by the "cardinal obligation to protect the welfare and integrity of the individual with whom he was working" (Schwitzgebel & Schwitzgebel, 1980,

p. 136). If we were to apply his behavior to the ethical standards of the American Psychological Association as well, he would clearly be in violation of principles regarding responsibility, competence, moral and legal standards, and especially principles which relate to the protection of the welfare of the client.

In general, most researchers agree that such sexual involvement with clients takes dangerous and unfair advantage of clients. Such actions, in my opinion, abuse the special privileges and trust inherent in a helping relationship. The sanctity of such relationships should preclude the possibility of invasion of privacy, undue influence. dangerousness and the like. Unfortunately, as we are so often reminded, the disparity between the ideal and the real is often great.

Perhaps Kleinhaus was correct when he said, "hypnosis should absolutely not be included in the category of interesting, amusing or entertaining phenomena because of the potential psychological dangers and prolonged suffering it may bring to even apparently balanced individuals" (Kleinhaus, 1979, p. 224).

This matter could greatly be amended by public service announcements of an educative nature. The same should hold true regarding the general practice of medicine and psychotherapy. People should be informed and educated about the potential dangers of these professions. Of course, by the same token it would be worthwhile to consider the possibility of educating the public regarding the potential benefits of such activities.

High standards of professional training should be required and maintained to provide assurance to the consumer that services of the professional they may seek are represented by high levels of competency. Claims made regarding the effectiveness of hypnotic treatment should be supported by some sort of empirical validation. With regard to hypnosis, most authors cited agree that, at present, there has been little in the way of such empirical research conducted which might highlight the basic tenets and assumptions underlying its practice.

REFERENCES

Conn, J. Is hypnosis really dangerous? *The International Journal of Clinical and Experimental Hypnosis,* 1972, *20*(2), 61–79.

Freedman, A., Kaplan, H., & Sadock, B. *Modern Synopsis of the Textbook of Psychiatry II.* Baltimore: The Williams and Wilkins Co., 1976.

Kleinhaus, M., Dreyfuss, D., Beran, B., Goldberg, T., & Azikri, D. Some affect-effects of stage hypnosis: A case of psychopathological manifestations, *The International Journal of Clinical and Experimental Hypnosis,* 1979, *27*(3), 219-226.

Kline, M. the production of antisocial behavior through hypnosis: New clinical data, *The International Journal of Clinical and Experimental Hypnosis,* 1972, *20*(2), 80-94.

Lichtenstein, E. *Psychotherapy: Approaches and Applications.* Monterey CA: Brooks/Cole Publishing Company, 1980.

Orne, M. Can a hypnotized subject be compelled to carry out otherwise unacceptable behavior?, *The Journal of Clinical and Experimental Hypnosis,* 1972, *20*(2), 101-117.

Perry, C. Hypnotic coercion and compliance to it: A review of evidence presented in a legal case, *The International Journal of Clinical and Experimental Hypnosis,* 1979, *27*(3), 187-218.

Schwitzgebel, R. & Schwitzgebel, R. *Law and Psychological Practice.* NY: John Wiley and Sons, 1980.

Watkins, J. Antisocial behavior under hypnosis: Possible or Impossible?, *The International Journal of Clinical and Experimental Hypnosis,* 1972, *20*(2), 95-100.

Wolberg, L. Hypnotherapy. In Areti, S. (Ed.), *American Handbook of Psychiatry, Volume 2.* NY: Basic Books, Inc., 1959.

Wolbert, L. *Hypnosis: Is it for you?* NY: Harcourt Brace Jovanovich, 1972.

The Ethics of Biofeedback

CHAPTER 13

JAMES P. LE CLAIR

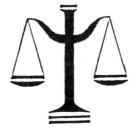

THE ETHICS OF BIOFEEDBACK

13

James P. LeClair

Biofeedback represents a relatively recent treatment innovation within the field of psychology which has received a good deal of attention from both the general public and numerous researchers/therapists. Biofeedback techniques involve a number of different procedures "wherein some aspect of an individual's physiological functioning is systematically monitored and fed back to that individual, typically in the form of an auditory or visual signal. The individual's task then is to modify that signal in order to change that physiological function or process in some way" (Rimm & Masters, 1979, p. 441).

Such procedures have utilized many different types of feedback (muscle tension, skin-surface temperature, galvanic skin response, brain wave activity, blood pressure, heart rate) and have been applied to a wide range of human difficulties including physical, emotional, and psychosomatic disorders (Brown, 1977).

Since biofeedback first achieved widespread popularity in the 1960s, a great amount of publicity has been generated with regard to the potential of such treatments (Yates, 1980). Yet, in the midst of this attention, one aspect that has received insufficient exploration is the question of ethical concerns as applied to this area. In this regard, there seems to be a curious lack within the professional literature, of articles addressing such vital issues. As such, it is the purpose of this paper to explore many of the salient issues within the field of biofeedback as they relate to important questions of ethics. However, rather than provide lengthy discussions with regard to such areas as confidentiality, patient rights, deception, research procedures, etc., which apply to the field of psychology as a whole, including biofeedback, this paper will instead concentrate on a sampling of the more important ethical issues which appear unique to the area of biofeedback.

Professional Issues

One of the unique characteristics of biofeedback has to do with its applicability to areas involving both mind and body. It has been found useful in dealing with aspects of both organic illnesses and psychological problems. In fact, biofeedback procedures themselves seem to represent an uncommon blend of both medical and psychological techniques. Because biofeedback can affect both physiological and psychological functions, with each in turn capable of influencing the other, a very real ethical problem often arises over who should assume responsibility for the patient's total well-being relative to both medical and psychological aspects. This dilemma is heightened somewhat by background differences between medically and psychologically trained practitioners of biofeedback (Brown, 1977).

The question of whether biofeedback rightfully belongs within the domain of medicine or psychology is a very complex one which is still the subject of much controversy. Yet it would seem that the best ethical solution to this problem, from the standpoint of the patient, should involve a partnership between the two fields.

Perhaps Shapiro and Surwit put it best when they said:

> The need for medical participation in any biofeedback case is both an ethical and legal responsibility of the psychological practitioner. Conversely, it is also the ethical responsibility of a physician who wishes to employ biofeedback in treatment to consult with a psychologist for the behavioral aspects of the proposed therapy. Medical training usually does not provide the in-depth knowledge of behavioral variables of which the practitioner must be cognizant in order for training to be successful. Therefore, the use of biofeedback in therapy for various physiological disorders should be a collaborative endeavor involving both medical and behavioral specialists (Shapiro & Surwit, 1979, p. 350).

Another area of ethical concern stems in part from the somewhat exaggerated and naive claims made for biofeedback in the news media which have accompanied the growth of this new field. Such reports have resulted in widespread sensationalism and a high degree of misinformation in the general public as to the true status of biofeedback. The fact is that, while biofeedback has been found useful in some situations, it has proven relatively ineffective in others, or at least no better than alternate forms of treatment (Wickramasekera, 1976). This field has also suffered from a lack of rigorous research and experimentation which has contributed to the "mystique" surrounding such techniques.

In addition, questions arise about record keeping, about the type of biofeedback most applicable to a specific disorder, about evaluations over effectiveness, and so on (Brown, 1977). Ethically it would seem expedient for practitioners in this area to not only employ more substantial and well-controlled studies in determining the value of biofeedback but also to continue disseminating more accurate pictures of the current state-of-affairs within this field as well as actively challenging the more dubious claims for effectiveness which seem to appear regularly in the news media (Shapiro, 1973).

Biofeedback Practitioners and Their Subjects

Since there is much we do not know in this area, the therapist should be cautious with regard to claims made for biofeedback. In dealing with clients the usual procedures pertaining to informed consent should always be adhered to and the client should be made fully aware of alternate treatment methods for particular maladies. A complete psychophysiological profile should be obtained along with appropriate medical work-ups and consultation. The patient's fears and beliefs should be explored as they apply to biofeedback and the specifics of goals and treatment should be discussed and mutually agreed upon (Gaarder & Montgomery, 1977).

From an ethical standpoint the therapist should be knowledgeable both with regard to possible problems that may arise in treatment as well as with regard to instances where biofeedback might be inappropriate. According to Fuller, such problem areas might involve the following:

(a) concurrent medication, or premature withdrawal from medication, especially in hypertension, diabetes, and epilepsy; (b) age, in that hypotension can occur in deep relaxation; (c) improper training, such as low-frequency brain-wave training in epilepsy, unilateral electrode placement in bruxism, or improper and unbalanced target sites for muscle reeducation; (d) psychosis, in which the biofeedback instruments may be woven into the delusional framework of control of the mind, or where the relaxation experience may enhance dissociative feelings; (e) cardiac dysfunction, such as cardiac arrhythmias, treatment of which is best accomplished with the life-support equipment available in a hospital coronary-care unit; and (f) insufficient arousal, in that the client should achieve a full state of awareness following biofeedback and relaxation procedures before leaving the office (Fuller, 1978, p. 45).

It is vitally important in this area to set realistic goals with patients. Many individuals who seek biofeedback training may themselves be victims of the early optimistic publicity surrounding this field and may be seeking the "miracle" of biofeedback. For example, it would be extremely unrealistic for a person suffering from stroke paralysis to expect a complete return of functions to pre-stroke levels through the use of biofeedback. Thus it is contingent upon biofeedback therapists to both educate patients and aid them in the setting of realistic goals (Yates, 1980).

Another aspect concerns the importance of constantly evaluating and following up on the progress of individual biofeedback subjects. Information as to the effectiveness of the program should be made readily available to the patient on a regular basis. Also, ethically it is the duty of the therapist to terminate biofeedback training when it becomes apparent that the patient is not benefiting from the experience (Yates, 1980). The degree to which such values are stressed in this field is made clear by Schwartz when he stated, ". . . the non-evaluative use of biofeedback in certain clinical settings is not only irresponsible and potentially unsafe, but is counter to the basic premise regarding the role of information and feedback in the development and maintenance of stable self-regulation" (Schwartz, 1979, p. 274).

Competency Issues

The area of therapist training and competency in the use of biofeedback has received increasing attention in recent years, especially in view of the fact that there are so few laws governing the use of biofeedback. However, in general, a potential biofeedback therapist should ideally be a licensed health professional (i.e., physician, psychologist, physical therapist, etc.) who has expertise in certain key areas (Fuller, 1978).

The first area is that of psychology, so as to be able to design appropriate methodologies and apply relevant psychological strategies in implementing biofeedback programs. Such training would be important in dealing with many situations, as in the case of patients who may be using their symptoms for secondary gain. A second area of expertise should be relative to the field of physiology and physical medicine so as to have a working knowledge and understanding of the biological response system being affected by biofeedback training.

In this regard, for example, it would be important for the therapist to realize the dangers of relying upon forehead EMG measures relative to frontalis activity or anxiety estimates. Also, it would seem logical that in such situations as migraine, in order to adequately treat it with biofeedback, some knowledge of its physiology is necessary. The third area of expertise should involve specific biofeedback training as well as a knowledge of electronics so as to be aware of the workings and safety characteristics of the instrumentation being utilized (Gratchel & Price, 1979).

Another area would involve the ability of the prospective therapist to demonstrate competency on certification examinations as provided by various biofeedback societies. The final area basically involves having had personal experience in effecting the same type of physiological processes which will later be expected from clients. In this regard, there seems to be a feeling that in order to be fully comprehended, biofeedback must actually be experienced by the prospective therapist (Fuller, 1978).

Obviously, no matter what one's background, weekend workshops hardly prepare an individual with the expertise needed to adequately treat people with biofeedback. The Biofeedback Society of California has adopted the following training guidelines:

Approved training programs provide 120 hours in the following categories: (a) didactic instruction, which provides basic information on biofeedback, including theory, use of instruments, research, clinical applications and procedures, and relaxation techniques (40 hours required); (b) case studies, which focus on syndromes and clinical cases, procedures, problems, contraindications, home practice, ethics, and placebo effects (10 hours); (c) personal training so that trainees gain personal biofeedback experience with instruments of at least four different types (25 hours) (d) clinical experience in working with clients (30 hours); and (3) supervision of clinical experience and other technical issues of biofeedback (15 hours) (Fuller, 1978, p. 47).

At the present time there appears to be many practitioners who lack the training and knowledge implied in the foregoing discussion. This raises a number of ethical, legal, and medical questions in that failure to rule out certain medical problems (i.e., headaches resulting from a brain tumor, etc.) or the altering of certain physiological functions can result in dangerous outcomes. Careful monitoring of new innovations in biofeedback have often been lacking in the past and it would seem that some form of "watchdog" committee or agency should be developed in order to insure a preponderance of adequately trained and compatent biofeedback clinicians and researchers (Gratchel & Price, 1979).

More and more such responsibilities seem to be falling upon the various biofeedback organizations which have arisen in recent years. This topic will be discussed further in a later section of this paper. For the time being, however, suffice it to say that biofeedback practitioners have an ethical responsibility to police their own field and report to the appropriate agency or organization any instances of improperly trained therapists or inappropriate biofeedback applications of which they may have knowledge. They also have an ethical and professional obligation to keep abreast of the rapidly accumulating amount of research which appears regularly in various journals (Gaarder & Montgomery, 1977).

Another area of ethical concern has to do with the increasing use of aides or technicians to assist therapists in their daily schedules. Often such aides become involved directly with patients as in monitoring and sometimes lengthy biofeedback sessions or in answering patient questions. It goes without saying that the professional therapist has an ethical responsibility to adequately supervise such paraprofessionals and in other ways provide for their appropriate training (Gaarder & Montgomery, 1977).

Biofeedback Machines

Biofeedback machines have been on the market now for several years and have been the source of much misinformation. Extravagant and unfounded claims have permeated this area while the quality and availability of such instruments continue to vary widely. Presently, such devices are considered "multiple-use" items. "If such a device is used, for example, to treat migraine headache, then it may be classified as a medical device. If the instrument, however, is used to enhance thought processes or teach techniques of control of emotional responses (without being used to treat a disease or to substantially affect a health-related physiological function), then it may be classified as a psychological device" (Switzgebel & Schwitzgebel, 1980, p. 140).

The distinction between medical and psychological biofeedback devices is often ambiguous but in one way or another such machines are now usually subject to regulations by at least one of three federal agencies: the Food and Drug Administration (FDA), the Federal Trade Commission, or the Consumer Product Safety Commission (Schwitzgebel & Schwitzgebel, 1980). Perhaps the most active agency in this area is the FDA. In most cases, it appears that biofeedback machines are considered medical devices and, as such, are subject to FDA requirements in regard to performance levels, safety and effectiveness levels, and labeling standards. The relatively recent development of portable biofeedback devices with built-in computer modules for quantifying and displaying information, aside from increasing the range of applications within the field, has added significantly to the work of these agencies (Schwartz, 1979).

In spite of such regulatory agencies, misleading advertising, faulty machines, etc., still tend to be much in evidence. Biofeedback therapists have an ethical responsibility to report to the appropriate agency any such instances so that corrective action can be promptly and efficiently undertaken. Even in the best of machines, however, periodic equipment failure occurs or false feedback can often distort and adversely affect treatment. An example of this is reported by Gatchel & Price, who indicated that: "We once witnessed a dramatic demonstration of the reduction in forehead temperature by one patient, over five degrees Fahrenheit in the space of a few minutes. It turned out that the tape holding the thermistor in place had gradually worked itself loose, making the thermistor's connection with the skin increasingly tenuous" (Gratchel & Price, 1979, p. 232).

False signals can occur for many reasons and include such aspects as weak batteries, poor electrode application and placement, electrical interference, broken wires, etc. Such concerns dictate that the therapist have adequate training and familiarity with biofeedback devices so as to determine whether the signal change is resulting from the equipment and preparation, or whether they reflect accurate physiological alterations. Adequate knowledge of physiological mechanisms is also important. Needless to say, biofeedback practitioners should closely follow the manufacturer's specifications and directions that accompany the machine and should be thoroughly familiar with its operation prior to actual therapeutic use (Gaarder & Montgomery, 1977).

The present discussion on biofeedback machines could go on in many directions and encompass many different aspects. However, the bottom-line in all of these areas involves a therapist's understanding and familiarity with the electronic components of such devices. At this point it should be noted that in cases involving physical or mental injury due to faulty biofeedback equipment (i.e., shocks), it is usually the manufacturer or seller who must bear the brunt of liability unless it can be proven that the therapist failed to properly maintain the instrument, or in other ways exceeded manufacturer specifications. In the actual purchase of machines, therapists are usually well-advised to select instruments which have met basic requirements from an appropriate regulatory agency; i.e., FDA (Schwitzgebel & Schwitzgebel, 1973).

On another topic, numerous guidelines presently exist for the utilization of biofeedback machines in both clinical practice and experimentation to which therapists should generally adhere. Such procedures usually involve aspects of informed consent, patient rights, instances when regulatory or supervisory agencies should be contacted, and so on. The reader interested in these aspects is referred to Schwitzgebel and Schwitzgebel (1980) for a more complete description.

On a final note, in a personal communication with the FDA, it was learned that some biofeedback machines are restricted relative to their availability to the general public. This is determined usually by the complexity of the machine and its intended purpose (i.e., medical, psychological, etc.). As an example certain biofeedback machines, classified as medical devices, are often subject to regulations from the various State Boards of Medical Examiners. The potential of misuse of biofeedback machines is obviously a key determinant in any decision to restrict sales. However, as such instruments continue to be refined and the distinction between medical, psychological, and other uses blurs, there arises potential future difficulties relative to the sale of such devices which undoubtedly can have many ethical repercussions; i.e., undue restrictions of biofeedback use, etc. (Brown, 1977).

Biofeedback Organizations and Miscellaneous Areas

The main organization in the area of biofeedback appears to be the Biofeedback Society of America. This professional group has chapters in many states and has taken upon itself the responsibilities for policing the area of biofeedback. This association has taken the lead in grappling with the many problem areas within the field and has helped establish guidelines relative to such areas as ethics, training, competency, and so on. It has also taken the lead in shaping both legislation and regulations aimed at tightening what in the past has been a loosely knit field. Relative to certification (which should not be confused with state the association (the BSA) has established testable competency levels for individuals involved in biofeedback which are designed to assess individual's basic understanding and use of the techniques in this area (Fuller, 1978).

As previously mentioned, there are few actual laws regulating the use of biofeedback. In general, states tend to simply license particular professions such as psychology, medicine, etc., and in most cases it is up to the individual profession to determine whether biofeedback is included under that licensure. In this regard, the 1977 Psychology Licensure Act, pertaining to the state of California, included the area of biofeedback. Certain federal legislation (Medical Devices Amendment) has indicated that biofeedback practitioners must be licensed providers, thus leaving it up to the individual states to determine which professions are actually covered. Such legislation as this obviously has had an effect on curtailing the number of untrained biofeedback therapists. While this has cut down on the problem, it has not eliminated it and thus, continued ethical vigilance would seem to be necessary (Fuller, 1978).

There are two other areas involving some offshoots of ethical issues which are currently receiving attention and therefore will be briefly mentioned at this time. The first area involves insurance payments for biofeedback services. Confusion seems apparent, in that different insurance companies react in different ways to biofeedback training. Some consider such training as appropriate to treatments within each of the professions (medicine, psychology, physical therapy) and some do not, utilizing instead a separate billing category. Some consider biofeedback as part of psychiatric services and cover it only to the degree to which psychiatric services are covered. Some have difficulty in deciding who are considered eligible providers or what type of disorders should legitimately be covered under biofeedback auspices. Difficulties are also apparent relative to the utilization of paraprofessionals. Some will reimburse for such services while others do so only if the professional directly administers the treatment (Fuller, 1978).

The second related area involves malpractice insurance. Here questions again arise with regard to the vulnerability of the professional utilizing technicians. Most professionals appear to be covered under policies which include clauses for biofeedback use. At any rate, relative to such a possible contingency, Fuller indicates that it is important for the biofeedback therapist:

> . . . (a) to be aware of the precautions and contraindications; (b) to be cautious as to the treatment services provided; (c) to be conservative as to the results claimed; (d) to have adequate high-risk conditions; and (e) to have expert legal advice in the development of a practice (Fuller, 1978, p. 46).

Concluding Comments

The foregoing discussion of ethical and legal concerns in biofeedback is not exhaustive, nor could it be within the confines of this brief chapter. Rather, the focus was more upon those elements which seemed to surface frequently within the biofeedback literature. If any one thing stands out clearly, it is the fact that, with few exceptions, most of the issues and principles in biofeedback tend to be quite similar to those experienced at one time or another in other areas of psychology as well as in other professions.

Many of the issues currently surfacing within the field stem in part from the relatively recent birth of this technique, while others are the result of the rather unique treatment methods which highlight its distinctive character. That this new approach to treatment offers promise in many areas is without question. Indeed there seems to be something inherently appealing and ethically pleasing about this nonpharmacological, noninvasive means of treatment which stresses such concepts as self-control, self-help, self-responsibility, and self-regulation of bodily processes (Peper, Pelliter, & Tandy, 1979). Yet such treatment techniques suffer from the same problems which characterize most of the other treatment approaches within psychology, inconclusive evidence as to both actual effectiveness and actual superiority over alternate treatment methods relative to many disorders (Yates, 1980). Related unanswered questions involve the influence of individual difference variables in biofeedback, the carry-over effects of biofeedback training in the absence of direct feedback, and so on, all of which in combination can give rise to what Shapiro and Surwit term the "question of economy":

> How much time and effort, on the part of both the patient and the practitioner, are needed to obtain a clinically useful result? Even if biofeedback techniques can be shown to be therapeutically effective, what patient would opt for a costly, time-consuming training course if equal therapeutic benefit could be obtained from a pill? . . . Unless the side effects of the medication are serious or the efficacy of biofeedback is shown to be superior to that of medication, it seems unlikely that biofeedback will be considered as a treatment of choice (Shapiro & Surwit, 1979, p. 32).

Along the same lines, one can ask similar justification questions relative to the advantages of biofeedback training for general anxiety versus the more traditional and somewhat simpler relaxation methods. The same questions arise with regard to many other areas of biofeedback training as well, all of which brings up another ethical question over the degree to which such techniques should actually be utilized at this point in therapeutic settings, without more conclusive outcome results than presently exist. This is a question which spans not only biofeedback but the entire area of psychology as well, all of which should give one pause to wonder.

By the above discussion, I do not imply that a moratorium should be placed upon all therapeutic treatments within the field of psychology, including that of biofeedback. Rather, what is needed are more in-depth and well-controlled studies which will allow for a better evaluation and understanding of the true merits of each of our treatment methods. In the meantime it would seem that our ethical responsibilities could best be served by more insight on the part of each of us into our professional limitations at this point in time, both with regard to ourselves and to our treatment techniques.

REFERENCES

American Psychological Association. *Ethical Standards of Psychologists.* Washington DC: American Psychological Association, 1979.

Brown, B. *Stress and the Art of Biofeedback.* NY: Bantam Books, Inc., 1977.

Fuller, G. Current status of biofeedback in clinical practice, *American Psychologist,* January 1978, 39–48.

Gaarder, K. & Montgomery, P. *Clinical Biofeedback: A Procedural Manual.* Baltimore: Williams & Wilkins Company, 1977.

Gratchel, R. & Price, K. (Eds.). *Clinical Applications of Biofeedback: Appraisal & Status.* NY: Pergamon Press, 1979.

Peper, E., Pelletier, K., & Tandy, B. Biofeedback training: Holistic and transpersonal frontiers, in E. Peper, S. Ancoli, M. Quinn (Eds.), *Mind/Body Integration.* NY: Plenum Press, 1979.

Rimm, D. & Masters, J. *Behavior Therapy, 2nd Ed.* NY: Academic Press, Inc., 1979.

Schwartz, G. Research and feedback in clinical practice: A commentary on responsible biofeedback therapy, in J. Basmajian, *Biofeedback: Principles and Practice for Clinicians.* Baltimore: Williams & Wilkins Company, 1970.

Schwitzgebel, R. & Schwitzgebel, R. *Psychotechnology: Electronic Control of Mind and Behavior.* NY: Holt, Rinehart and Winston, Inc., 1973.

Schwitzgebel, R. & Schwitzgebel, R. *Law and Psychological Practice.* NY: John Wiley & Sons, Inc., 1980.

Shapiro, D. Recommendations of Ethics Committee regarding biofeedback techniques and instrumentation: Issues of public and professional concern, *Psychophysiology*, 1973, *10*(5), 533–535.

Shapiro, D. & Surwit, R. Learned control of physiological function and disease, in E. Peper, S. Ancoli, & M. Quinn, *Mind/Body Integration*. NY: Plenum Press, 1979.

Wicramasekera, I. *Biofeedback, Behavior Therapy and Hypnosis*. Chicago: Nelson-Hall, 1976.

Yates, A. *Biofeedback and the Modification of Behavior*. NY: Plenum Press, 1980.

Ethics In Intelligence Testing

CHAPTER 14

PATRICIA M. ROYCE

ETHICS IN INTELLIGENCE TESTING

14

Patricia M. Royce

The influence of the intelligence test increased to immense proportions in the United States in the first six decades of this century and came to wield tremendous power over the lives of millions of people (Matarazzo, 1979; McClelland, 1973). Emphasis shifted after World War I from individual testing, which had its principal application in clinical settings where qualitative interpretations were made and decisions concerned only a few, to group testing which involved decisions for the many in institutional settings (Anastasi, 1976; Cronback, 1970).

Gradually it became apparent that such group intelligence tests could also be misused and misinterpreted, that they might not be truly effective in measuring that inherent ability the general public thought of as "intelligence," that they might not be equally fair to all people, that serious harm could come from placement in inappropriate educational programs, and that private information drawn from them could become public knowledge (Anastasi, 1976; Cronback, 1970; Flaugher, 1978; Schwitzgebel & Schwitzgebel, 1980; American Psychological Association, 1974).

Tests were often administered by untrained personnel but the results obtained from them were used nevertheless to screen out minorities, the culturally disadvantaged, and the handicapped from jobs and educational opportunities. School children were labeled, classified and identified (Buros, 1965) by IQ scores which were added to their cumulative folders and thereafter followed them from school to school (Sharp, 1972). A low IQ score placed an indelible stamp of inferiority on a child (Anastasi, 1976; Buros, 1965). Many youngsters were pigeonholed into academic and rigid lifetime molds. According to Dr. Benjamin Fine, "the caste system lived in IQ tests" (Fine, 1975, p. 1).

As early as 1965, Buros was laying the blame for IQ evils on this mass substitution of the group test for the more time-consuming but accurate individual test, and Guilford (1967) stated that it was alarming to contemplate what the exclusive use of answer sheet tests, which cannot assess creativity or motivation, and the effect these differences may have on scores, could do to the intellectual character of a nation. In 1964, as the implication of permanent status became more firmly attached to the IQ and the IQ battle raged, New York City stopped the use of group tests in its public schools.

In the past decade ethical questions have been raised, laws passed, and cases tried. The group intelligence test, a rough screening device at best (Sharp, 1972), has never been held in less esteem by the general public. Leading court cases have not held intelligence testing or ability grouping *per se* to be illegal, but they have held that the misuse of tests or grouping is illegal (Schwitzgebel & Schwitzgebel, 1980).

These same legal proceedings, however, while outlawing group intelligence tests in many cases, have effectively mandated the use of individual intelligence tests. A Federal Court in Philadelphia found, in 1972, that public education should be provided for all mentally retarded students, even those with the lowest IQ scores. Individual tests are required for the diagnosis of mental retardation in Pennsylvania, as well as most other states (Sharp, 1972). Other populations are also in need of special treatment or remediation—in mental health programs, special education classes, and individual education programs for physically handicapped children (Schwitzgebel & Schwitzgebel, 1980).

Society demands that psychologists classify, diagnose, and predict performance, and because it is recognized that measures of intelligence are responsible for a large part of the variance in such predictions (Vernon, 1978), the use of intelligence tests has now come full circle. Once more the individual IQ test has become an integral part of the assessment procedures required to make skilled placement decisions. Legal inquiry has sought to clarify the difference between the ethical use of tests in such decisions and their use for isolating individuals from educational and employment opportunities due to some presumed biological deficit (Schwitzgebel & Schwitzgebel, 1980), a use which is "a serious breach of professional ethics" (Deutsch et al., 1964, p. 144). The question has become then, not whether to use these tests, but rather, how to use them, effectively and ethically.

As Wechsler observed in 1971, it is not an inherent fault of the IQ test itself that incompetent people have misused it (Wechsler, 1971). Psychological assessment is a professional activity and it is more than mere psychological testing (Matarazzo, 1979). The ethical use of intelligence tests requires first a test administrator with an appropriate educational background, who is properly experienced and sufficiently trained and disciplined to follow all instructions and guidelines (Sattler, et al., 1978; Cleary, et al., 1975).

Test-givers must know the strengths of intelligence tests, but must also be aware of their limitations. Such tests measure only the subject's current status. IQ scores are an estimate of performance under a given set of circumstances—the score on a particular test at a particular time— and are subject to change. They cannot be interpreted as some absolute characteristic of the examinee or as something permanent and generalizable to all other circumstances (American Psychological Association, 1974; Sattler, 1974). Examiners must be cognizant also of their own strengths and limitations, their biases, and the effect their cultural backgrounds may have on the examinee and on their own diagnostic and prognostic inferences about that examinee (Ryan, 1980; Anastasi, 1976). Examiners must give the test under carefully controlled conditions and yet be able to draw out the best in their subject and remain sensitive to the level of the examinee's motivation during testing (Buros, 1965).

Examiners must know how to question and encourage, observe and record important behavioral responses and other data that are entirely dependent on their clinical experience and sagacity, and they must score the test properly—often a difficult and challenging task (Sattler, et al., 1978; Waite, 1961). Interpretation of the test results in each individual case is a highly complex and professional enterprise. Here too, examiners must have considerable training and experience. Subjects may obtain identical IQ scores but arrive at them in quite different ways, and that difference may be important (Matarazzo, 1979). Alternative interpretations of given scores must be considered and examiners must remember that an impression gained from a subject is useful, but it is not a scientific conclusion (Cronback, 1970; American Psychological Association, 1974). Examiners must be able to translate their findings into language that is not subject to misinterpretation by those for whom they provide it or those to whom it might become available (Garfield & Affleck, 1960). They are responsible also for maintaining confidentiality; they report test findings only to the subject (or to the parents, if it is a child), the referral agency (such as a clinic, a school, or a physician), the treatment team, and their own immediate supervisor (American Psychological Association, 1979).

The choice of a particular test must be considered carefully. The Examiners must insure that it is most appropriate for the individual case, is not outdated (Sharp, 1972), does not have serious defects, and is both reliable and valid. They must study the manual or other published information describing the development of the test and the rationale for it, the purposes and applications for which it was intended, and the characteristics of the population upon which it was standardized (Anastasi, 1976; American Psychological Association, 1979; Schwitzgebel & Schwitzgebel, 1980).

Most important of all, a psychologist must not use an individual intelligence test score *alone* to diagnose or predict. An IQ score can be a critical beginning datum, but, as Matarazzo stated, "it cannot be used in a vacuum" (Matarazzo, 1979, pp. 287–288).

IQ tests measure only a part of the broad spectrum of human abilities and before making a prediction of academic or employment success, or a diagnosis for clinical or placement purposes, examiners must evaluate a host of other capacities, such as motivation, adaptation to environment, or emotional problems, by other psychological and educational measures (Sattler, 1974; Fine, 1975; Garfield & Affleck, 1960). Intelligence tests represent only one source of data to be utilized in making decisions and "are not in themselves decision-making instruments" (Anastasi, 1976, p. 350). They serve as the bases for hypotheses that may prove to be the conclusions of further assessment.

The word "diagnosis" is used in several different ways—to describe individuals' observed style, to suggest inferences about their motivations and reactions to people and to tasks, or to place them in a category of psychiatric disorder. Although "diagnosis" refers to the present condition and "prediction" connotes a temporal estimate (Cronback, 1970), mental tests have an integral place in both areas. When an alert and trained clinician is in active contact with a person for the time required to administer a test, a great deal can be learned about that individual. Examiners collect data regarding the subject's mode of reaction, their special abilities or disabilities, and some indication of their personality traits (Matarazzo, 1979). These behavioral observations, the content of the subjects' answers, and the pattern of their subtest performance scores, when combined with the tester's experience and theoretical knowledge, suggest a much richer picture of the individual than a test score alone can convey (Cronback, 1970).

Ethical clinicians watch individual subtest results and individual answers; they are always sensitive to the non-cognitive factors which may affect intellectual performance (Garfield & Affleck, 1960). If they observe anxious, stressful behavior which seriously interferes with performance on certain types of tests which require careful observation and concentration, they consider that fact in their interpretations (Anastasi, 1976; American Psychological Association, 1974). A subtest that may be scored only for correctness and speed, also provides the examiner with much information about the subject's natural style of problem-solving (Sharp, 1972).

Significant leads may emerge from the form as well as the content of test responses. Answers may reveal disturbances of thinking and emotional processes (Cronbach, 1970). Responses should be recorded verbatim therefore, with interpretive comments which, even though speculative at the time, can be considered later in relation to other data (Waite, 1961).

Ethical examiners also note what is needed to help individuals do their best—what must be done to secure the examinee's attention, what must be repeated, what extraneous activities must be prevented (Sattler, 1974). Administration procedures can be flexible enough to encourage the subject to participate without jeopardizing test standardization; extra time can be allowed for establishing rapport; ambiguous answers can be questioned additionally to insure more accurate scoring (Sattler, et al., 1978).

Freeman (1976) has shown that certain behavioral techniques can be used to facilitate the testing of children. Examiners can also add the "testing of limits" procedure after the completion of the test, a practice which is of particular use in the case of the mentally retarded where behavior is as important as test scores in diagnosis. Ascertaining the number of cues they must give before the subject can answer a question, discovering the problem-solving methods used, and re-administering the test without time limits all add significantly to the amount of knowledge gained about the examinee (Sattler, 1974).

Studies have shown that when individual intelligence test scores and behaviors are carefully examined, analyzed, and evaluated by an ethical examiner the results can be of great diagnostic and predictive value, and may not have been utilized sufficiently in many cases. Lambert reported in 1978 that the Wechsler Intelligence Scale for Children, Revised (WISC-R) was an important tool for discovering abilities in mentally retarded children that might not otherwise have been discerned (Lambert, 1978).

Robert Gordon (1978), who was himself helped out of an orphanage and into eventual professorship at Johns Hopkins University by IQ tests, stated that intelligence tests have been the greatest finders of talented children who might otherwise have been neglected and overlooked, and that they may actually have kept more children out of classes for the mentally retarded than they ever put in them. Besides calling for definite placement in special education programs, objective evaluation of an intelligence test may call for a child to remain in a regular classroom with later reassessment, if indicated (Buros, 1975).

According to Matarazzo (1979), there is now beginning evidence that measured intelligence may be useful in the diagnosis of potential school failure or dropout and that IQ tests can thus alert teachers and parents to the need for preventive intervention, tailored to the unique requirements of each youngster, at a very early age. Sattler (1974) also saw IQ tests as a valid index of what needs to be done for a particular child, the place to begin to bring the child up to maximum effectiveness.

Results of a longitudinal study conducted in The Netherlands showed that intelligence test profiles of dyslexic college students differed markedly from those of normal students, making classification of dyslexia or non-dyslexia with a certainty of 80 percent (Kuipers & Weggerlaar, 1978).

Gift, Strauss, and Ritzler (1978) found that level of intellectual functioning was still often overlooked as a variable of major import for diagnosis and planning in the care of hospitalized psychiatric patients. A review of the literature supports the conclusion that IQ tests are of prognostic value with neurotic patients (Waite, 1961), with autistic and schizophrenic children (Freeman, 1976; Sattler, 1974), and in the prediction of vocational success of psychiatric outpatients (Clarizio, 1979; Webster, 1979).

Intelligence has never been regarded by society as a psychological concept only. It has always been a "precious, tenaciously guarded social concept" (Matarazzo, 1979, p. 22). IQ tests were oversold in the beginning and capabilities they never had were attributed to them (Sharp, 1972). Now a broader view of intelligence is emerging. It is no longer seen as a capacity but as a behavioral trait that is highly dependent on past learning, but is not a fixed trait (Cleary, 1975).

Intelligence tests are now considered as maps on which it is possible to locate individuals' present position in order to facilitate an understanding of them and to assist in effective planning for their optimal development. Thus ethical and responsible utilization of an intelligence test by a fully qualified clinician, and with the informed consent of examinees, can help those individuals move from their present position, no matter at what relative level, toward the attainment of their full potential.

REFERENCES

American Psychological Association. *Standards for Educational and Psychological Tests.* Washington DC, 1974.

American Psychological Association, *Ethical Standards of Psychologists.* Washington DC, 1979.

Anastasi, A. *Psychological Testing, 4th Ed.* NY: Macmillan Publishing Co., Inc. 1976.

Buros, O. Decline and fall of group intelligence testing, *Teaching College Record,* October, 1965, cited by E. Sharp, *The IQ Cult.* NY: Coward, McCann & Geoghegan, 1972.

Buss, W. What procedural due process means to a school psychologist: A dialogue, *Journal of School Psychology,* Winter 1975, *XIII,* 317–323.

Clarizio, H. In defense of the IQ test, *School Psychology Digest,* Winter 1979, *XIII,* 79–88.

Cleary, A., Humphreys, L., Kendrick, S., & Wesman, A. Educational uses of tests with disadvantaged students, *American Psychologist,* January 1975, *XXX,* 15–41.

Cronback, L. *Essentials of Psychological Testing, 3rd Ed.* NY: Harper & Row, 1970.

Deutsch, M., Fishman, J., Kogan, L., North, R., & Whiteman, M. Guidelines for testing minority group children, *Journal of Social Issues,* 1964, *XX*(2), 129–145.

Fine, B. *The Stranglehold of the IQ.* Garden City NY: Doubleday & Company, Inc., 1975.

Flaugher, R. The many definitions of test bias, *American Psychologist,* July 1978, *XXXIII,* 671–679.

Freedman, A., Kaplan, H., & Saddock, B. *Modern Synopsis of Comprehensive Testbook of Psychiatry: II.* Baltimore: The William & Wilkins Co., 1980.

Freeman, B. Evaluating autistic children, *Journal of Pediatric Psychology,* 1976, *I*(3), 18–21.

Garfield S., & Affleck, D. A study of individuals committed to a state home for the retarded who were later released as not mentally defective, *American Journal of Mental Deficiency,* March 1960, *LXIV*(5), 907–915.

Gift, T., Strauss, J., & Ritzler, B. The failure to detect low IQ in psychiatric assessment, *American Journal of Psychiatry,* March 1978, *CXXV*(3), 345–349.

Gordon, R. Quoted in C. Holden, California Court Is Forum for Latest Round in IQ Debate, *Science,* September 1978, *CCI,* 1106–1109.

Guilford, J. *The Nature of Human Intelligence.* NY: McGraw-Hill Book Company, 1967.

Kuipers, C. & Weggelaar, C. Myklebust's cognitive structure hypothesis for 91 dyslexic students of Delft University of Technology, *Journal of Consulting and Clinical Psychology,* December 1977, *XLV*(6), 1178–1179.

Lambert, N. Quoted in Constance Holden, California Court Is Forum for Latest Round in IQ Debate, *Science,* September 1978, *CCI,* 1106–1109.

Matarazzo, J. *Wechsler's Measurement and Appraisal of Adult Intelligence, 5th Ed.* NY: Oxford University Press, 1979.

McClelland, D. Testing for competence rather than for intelligence, *American Psychologist,* January 1973, *XXVIII*(1), 1–14.

Ryan, M. Class Lecture, United States International University. San Diego California, October 9, 1980.

Sattler, J. *Assessment of Children's Intelligence.* Philadelphia: W. B. Saunders Company, 1974.

Sattler, J., Andres, R., Squire, L., Wisely, R., & Maloy, C. Examiner scoring of ambiguous WISC-R responses, *Psychology in the Schools,* October 1978, *XVI*(4), 486–489.

Schwitzgebel, R. & Schwitzgebel, R. *Law and Psychological Practice.* NY: John Wiley & Sons, 1980.

Sharp, E. *The IQ Cult.* NY: Coward, McCann & Geoghegan, 1972.

Vernon, P. Recent attacks on the concept of intelligence, *International Review of Applied Psychology,* October 1975, *XXIV*(2), 93–98.

Waite, R. The intelligence test as a psychodiagnostic instrument, *Journal of Projective Techniques*, March 1961, *XXV*(1), 90–102.

Webster, R. Utility of the WAIS in predicting vocational success of psychiatric patients, *Journal of Clinical Psychology,* January 1979, *XXV(1), 111–116.*

Wechsler, D. Intelligence: Definition, theory, and the IQ. In R. Cancro (Ed.), *Intelligence: Genetic and Environmental Influences.* NY: Grune and Stratton, 1971.

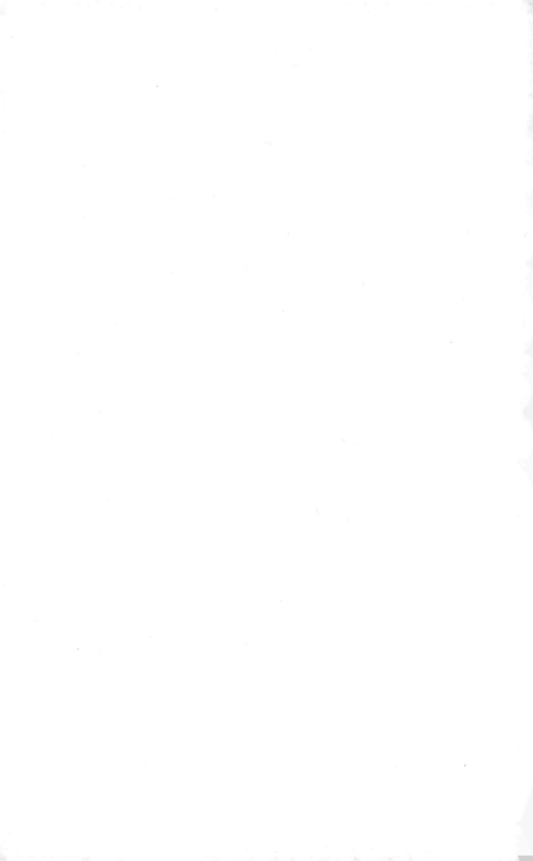

An Ethical Dilemma: The Needs Of The Client Versus Those Of The Military Organization

CHAPTER 15

PAUL L. CLACK

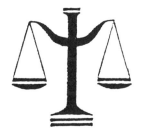

AN ETHICAL DILEMMA: THE NEEDS OF THE CLIENT VERSUS THOSE OF THE MILITARY ORGANIZATION

15

Paul L. Clack

In recent years professional issues have rapidly forged their way to a position of top priority in not only the medical field, but in the fields of psychology, social work, and other "helping professions." In the past, the American Psychological Association (APA), as a scientific organization, took a neutral stance on political, social, and professional issues. With hindsight, this appears to have been an antiquated position which hampered the development of psychology for years (Congdon, 1979, p. 1).

To combat undue legal restrictions for the profession, in 1974, the APA created a political advocacy arm, the Association for the Advancement of Psychology (AAP), which represents a dramatic turnaround from years past. This was a significant and necessary development if psychology was to avoid being legislated out of practice or, at best, having severe legal restrictions leveled against it.

Psychologists have come to realize the extreme power legislators have over the practice of psychology or any other profession. Unfortunately, psychology also came to realize that legislators knew little if anything about the role of psychologists and other mental health practitioners in delivering mental health services. The AAP was ushered in to fight for the professional independence of psychology since, for years physicians had collaborated with psychiatry to exclude psychologists from funding and insurance programs by requiring physician referral, and by successfully squashing any legislation designed to offer the professional independence psychologists desired.

Malpractice suits have done much to focus the attention of the profession on legal statutes and ethical principles. The costs of malpractice insurance have opened many professional eyes, particularly in the fields of medicine and law. Psychologists have remained on the periphery of this dilemma for some years now. While the cost of malpractice insurance has remained quite low for psychologists, there has been an increasing number of law suits through the years, some for large sums of money. The plaintiff in a law suit can recover two types of damages: general damages and punitive damages. Punitive damages, also called exemplary damages, are not covered by insurance policies, are in addition to general damages, and may be awarded where there has been a more willful disregard for a client's rights or safety (Campbell, 1977, p. 13). California, for instance, permits the award of exemplary damages in cases of "oppression, fraud, or malice, express or implied" committed by the defendant (see California Civil Code, Section 3294).

Establishing Ethical Standards

Ethical practices in psychology are concerned with the resolution of conflicts between varying social standards, practices and responsibilities rather than with the advocacy of ethical absolutes (Klin, Gurstein, Hymon, & Navron, 1979). Ethical standards are especially difficult to apply to new techniques in the helping professions. Therefore, one sees increasing concern with such issues in light of the proliferation of different types of group procedures as well as techniques for new and different therapeutic processes. In a sense, absolute ethical standards for psychologists have only been a minor problem since they appear to be so clear-cut. For example, it should be obvious that one does not set out to kill, maim, or, either physically or emotionally, injure one's clients. Thus, it is the more nebulous rules of behavior which often do not fall within the general society's framework for "good" and "bad" which present sticky ethical dilemmas and give rise to a need for the continued reexamination of ethical standards in psychology.

One must keep in mind that the application and interpretation of ethical standards is partially a function of the time and place in which they are applied. For example, only since the 1977 revision of the APA *Ethical Standard of Psychologists* is there a direct statement regarding "prohibition of sexual intimacies with a patient" (Klin, et al., 1979, p. 76). According to Klin and colleagues' research on ethical practices, as presented in *The Association for Advanced Training in the Behavioral Sciences*, there are several basic assumptions that should be kept in mind in considering ethical issues:

- Most people who do things that raise ethical questions basically have honest intentions and would be responsive to a questioning of their activities.

- A single change which may be good in and of itself may have negative consequences in a wider social system.

- Ethical issues are important not only for humane reasons but have considerable practical value in the long run. Professional activities that may offend the mores of the public and demonstrate what would be seen as ethical irresponsibility will eventually lose popular support which could be reflected in the loss of funding for mental health programs.

- We are only practicing our ethical responsibility when we are continually concerned about what is right in our professional functioning.

Indeed, there are certain prescribed standards which all mental health practitioners would adhere to almost intuitively, without having them delineated by an Ethics Committee. However, there remains the more nebulous and ill-defined realm or "gray area" in which practitioners, via their preferred therapeutic modality, have the option to exercise professional judgment in more unique situations where ethical absolutes do not exist. It is just this area where practitioners must practice caution in implementing non-standardized treatment, for if the client issues a complaint or sues for malpractice, whatever the reason or justification, the practitioner may be rendered accountable and would have to assume full professional and legal liability.

The Dilemma for Practitioners in the Military

Take note of the following two quotes:

"The ultimate client, if not the only client of the government attorney, psychologist, etc., is the advancement of the common good" (John R. Risher, Jr.)

"The administrator whom the professional advises. . . is the real client" (F. Trowbridge von Baur)

The problems inherent in attempting to provide instructions and/or guidelines for practitioners working in a military setting are epitomized by the above two conflicting statements. Federal employees who are mental health practitioners working in a military context face a real dilemma in determining professional ethical standards. This is the primary problem faced by those seeking to develop and provide instruction for the criteria of what professional responsibility will constitute.

A practitioner in a military setting may experience conflict in certain situations where the military code of justice takes precedence over the therapist's own professional ethics. The "mission" of any given military activity comes first. That is, if the rights of the active duty military person conflict with those of the organization, there may be a legal and ethical predicament for the mental health practitioner who attempts to adhere to his own professional code of ethics. Who is the final governing authority? The dilemma arises from the necessity to prioritize loyalties.

Presumably, for military persons there is no question as to where their allegiance falls. It is with their branch of service, the command structure, their "outfit." Recently there have been some questions raised regarding service members' right to free speech, collective bargaining via unionization, and other rights of expression.

According to Captain William S. Ostan, in an article entitled, "Unionization of the Military: Some Legal and Practical Considerations," in the *Military Law Review* (1977), "Collective bargaining by an installation commander with a union does not fit within the traditional American military structure."

Moreover, "The possibility of negotiating through collective bargaining a contract which could limit the ability of a commander to accomplish his mission poses a definite threat to national security. The fundamental need for obedience, discipline and unencumbered command structure makes it impossible for collective bargaining to operate in the American military structure without having a detrimental effect" (Ostan, 1977).

Arguably, no member of the armed forces can divide his allegiance between his commander and a union leader who may issue an order to strike or otherwise take part in a job action. Collective bargaining and military discipline may be incompatible in view of a military member's obligation, under principles of military discipline, to obey any lawful order of a superior. There appears to be no argument at this point, yet there is the question of where the military draws the line concerning personal freedom and the constitutionality of those rights. Beyond this, what other rights to privacy and/or confidentiality, for example, have been stripped away from military persons, given the circumstances where their command's mission takes precedence over individual freedom and rights. There are implications to this enigma that warrant examination.

A Constitutional Appraisal of First Amendment Rights

Three problem areas have been mentioned by Siemer, Hut, and Drake concerning this issue in their article, "Prohibition of Military Unionization: A Constitutional Appraisal," found in the *Military Law Review* (1977). They are as follows:

(1) Whether the First Amendment applies in the military context with more limited scope or force than in the civilian context.
(2) What substantive standards will be used to determine the constitutionality of the prohibition.
(3) What further constitutional limitations are imposed by the First Amendment overbreadth doctrine.

The threshold question is whether the First Amendment protects the freedoms of speech and association for those in the military. Some commentators who advocated an expansive view of the protection provided by the First Amendment were inclined to include the military in those "alien sectors" of society that "fall outside the area in which. . . freedom of expression must be maintained" (Emerson, 1964, p. 877). In *Parker v. Levy*, however, the Supreme Court held that while "military society has been a society apart from civilian society," and while "the rights of men in the armed forces must perforce be conditioned to meet certain overriding demands of discipline and duty," nevertheless "the members of the military are not excluded from the protection granted by the First Amendment" (Siemer, et al., 1977, p. 3).

Although the Court extended the protection of the First Amendment to military personnel, it also held that the unique character of the military mission justifies a narrower application of those protections than is afforded in a civilian context. The Courts have pointedly stated that:

The different character of the military community and of the military mission requires a different application of those first amendment protections. The fundamental necessity for obedience, and the consequent necessity for imposition of discipline, may render permissible within the military that which would be constitutionally impermissible outside it (Siemer, et al., 1977).

Given this injunction it appears that with the military environment individual rights may necessarily be subordinated to the overriding military mission and that the military may constitutionally prohibit conduct that is quite permissible in civilian life. The extent to which First Amendment protections are limited in the military context depends upon the substantive standards that the courts apply to determine when the government lawfully may prohibit or restrict expressive or associational conduct. Although the Supreme Court has never really formulated a general and cohesive mode of First Amendment analysis, it has followed primarily two related approaches. Under one approach the Court balances the importance of the government's interest in limiting speech or association against the individual's interest in the restricted speech or association. Under another approach, the Court looks in a more narrowly focused way to see whether there is a clear and present danger to a government interest. If such a danger is not present, the individual's interest takes precedence.

Under this analytical approach, the courts recognize that there will be frequent instances in which a statute or other government action will in some way burden expressive or associational conduct, and that neither right is absolute. The question whether the law or government action is constitutional, therefore, will turn on two determinations: first, a weighing of the respective interests of the individual and the government; and second, a review of the government's alternatives to see if any other approach could achieve the same result through less restrictive means (Siemer, et al., 1977, p. 7).

Parallels of Military Law to Patient Rights

This notion of "less restrictive means" follows closely the idea, in the mental health profession, of the "least restrictive treatment" for patients. With landmark decisions being made in the judicial system concerning the advocacy of patient rights, certain legal guidelines as well as ethical prescriptions for practitioners have been elucidated. How clearly these same guidelines may apply in practice, but not in theory, to practitioners working in a military context whose clientele consist of active duty military personnel is suspect. With the documentation by the courts, noted earlier, that "the military mission justifies a narrower application of those protections than is offered in a civilian context" (referring to First Amendment rights), it appears one could logically extrapolate this theme to include the idea that the protections concerning patient rights, such as right to treatment confidentiality, etc., one normally receives in the civilian community, would be viewed differently in the military community. That is, the military may justify a "narrower application" of these protections to its active duty personnel because the "mission" would justify it.

In late 1975 the Board of Ethical and Social Responsibility for Psychology was required to recommend official positions for the APA in matters of criminal justice involving psychology (Klin, et al., 1979, p. 88). Protecting the ethical rights of active duty service members is a dilemma similar to that which mental health practitioners in the private sector have of ensuring rights to patients. The primary dilemma to be dealt with by both camps at the beginning is to define whether their role is primarily to help the client (or in the case of the military, the service member), to further the system, or to serve the interests of society (or to advance the mission, in the military's case). However, the military commander is certain that the obligation is to the military, and the client's needs are subordinate.

The Board of Ethical and Social Responsibility for Psychology notes that most ethical norms prescribed for psychologists were derived from situations in which an individual freely contracts services with a private practitioner or voluntarily enters an experimental relationship. The difficulty is that such relationships fail to reflect the complexities that arise when an organizational third party, such as the military, the justice system, etc., makes competing claims on the loyalty of the practitioner, or in the case of the military, more specifically, the service member. Given these three concerns, i.e., the client, the system and society, the psychologist must be able to differentiate the kinds of obligations owed to each. Moreover, for practitioners working in a military context with active duty personnel constituting their clientele, the issue between the professionals' allegiance to the military system and their ethical responsibility to the client become further complicated. This situation creates still greater disparity when there are no specific directives that even vaguely establish a criterion for the legal and ethical practices and constraints for the practitioner working in this particular setting. Practitioners in this setting, it seems, must practice caution, weighing the variables carefully. The protections they can offer clients in the civilian community may differ, depending on the circumstances, from the protections they can offer service members in the military context as a "narrower application of these protections" related to military personnel.

Ethical Considerations for Practitioners in a Military Context

In order to resolve the dilemma posed by multiple loyalties, the Board of Ethical and Social Responsibility for Psychology indicated that "both the individual and the organization may be clients of the psychologist within that system" (Klin, et al., 1979, p. 88). The psychologist must establish different priorities in relation to the roles he is filling. In the role of a therapist providing treatment to persons who want to change their behavior, the psychologist, it would seem, should primarily be the agent of the individual. There may be other roles in which the system may be the client and not the individual, in a military context, e.g., assessment of performance for the purpose of selection to advancement of rate or rank, evaluation of risk a client may present if alcohol or drug addiction interfere or thwart essential performance of tasks related to assigned duties, etc. Whatever the case, it is most important that the practitioner working in the military setting inform the client of his/her responsibility with regard to confidentiality. This must be done *before* initiating diagnostic or therapeutic procedures. Regarding the practitioner's loyalty, the client should be fully informed of the existence of confidentiality, or lack of it, and of any circumstances that could trigger an exception to the agreed-upon principles. Then the individual at least has the option to decide what to reveal and what risks to take.

The essential issues regarding confidentiality excerpted from *Ethical Practices,* authored by Klin and associates included the following items:

- Information obtained about an individual in the course of teaching, practice, or investigation must be safeguarded by the psychologist.

- Information received in confidence can be revealed to certain other parties only after careful deliberation and when there is a clear and imminent danger to an individual or to society.
- In releasing information to others, only information that is germane to any questions being asked may be presented and only after informed consent has been obtained.
- Identities of individuals must be adequately disguised in presenting research findings.
- Confidentiality of professional communications about individuals must be maintained.
- The psychologist must make adequate provisions for the maintenance of confidentiality in the preservation and ultimate disposition of confidential records (Klin, et al., 1979).

Within a military context, demands may be placed on the practitioner that go beyond conditions of employment which would be considered reasonable in the civilian community. Safeguards must be exercised to recognize possible conflicts of interest that may arise. Although the conflict may be clarified, the difficulty here is the nature and direction of the loyalties on the part of the practitioner to the military organization or to the individual may not be clear.

Welfare of the Client

A primary concern of the ethical practitioner is to respect the client's integrity while protecting the welfare of society. This is an obligation of the psychologist. Impinging upon this process for psychologists, and particularly for practitioners working in a military or similar organizational environment, are the multiple loyalties and responsibilities inherent in the work of psychologists. This predicament is compounded in an organizational setting where allegiance is ill-defined. Difficulty will certainly arise where the interest of an institution or organization is in conflict with the interest of the individual or when sub-groups in an organization have opposing interests. It is essential for practitioners to be aware of their own commitments and clarify in a skillful manner the directions of their own responsibilities in a manner that will be congruent with the parameters of the structured organization.

212 Professional Ethics and Law in the Health Sciences

Another area, already mentioned, which needs perpetual review and clarification in considering the rights and welfare of the client are the difficult decisions inherent in the confidential nature of the practitioner's work. These dilemmas involve not only the personal convictions of psychologists but also the expectations of society expressed in its customs and laws, and in addition, the constraints the organization, military or otherwise, may impose.

Client welfare is most poignantly embraced by the ethical obligations of the psychologist to his client, to his profession, and to society. These obligations most typically come into focus as the practitioner attempts to establish with his client a rapport, an alliance, a therapeutic atmosphere in which the competent skills of the therapist are exercised in order that a professional service may be rendered.

Again, according to Klin and associates, the following are the general principles involved in the welfare of the client:

- The psychologist must be aware of conflicts of interest between what the psychologist does, the welfare and integrity of the client, and/or the organization for whom the psychologist works.
- The practitioner must inform parties of loyalties, responsibilities and what is to be done with the information obtained.
- The psychologist must present individuals in research with the freedom of choice with regard to participation.
- Sexual intimacies with clients constitutes unethical behavior.
- If the client becomes unable to continue paying fees, it is the psychologist's responsibility to try to help the client find alternative treatment services.
- It is expected that psychologists contribute a portion of their services for little or no financial return.
- When it is reasonably clear that the services being provided by the psychologist are not benefitting the client, services should be modified or terminated (Klin, et al., 1979).

As an employee of an organization, practitioners must come to understand the discrepancy between their own self-limiting ethical prescriptions that guide their professional conduct and the policies, mandates and parameters that provide the structure to the organization's definition of legal and ethical behavior for professionals working under the auspices of its administration. The balance may be delicate but it must be found.

Conclusions

It is incumbent upon responsible practitioners to become aware of legal and ethical issues that may affect their dissemination of professional services. Since the application and interpretation of ethical standards are partially a function of the time and place in which they are applied, it is critical for practitioners to be cognizant of the limitations imposed by these conditions, particularly those conditions of the organization that may alter ethical constraints. The difficulty in dealing with the confusion of this discrepancy between ethical standards is accentuated further for the practitioner in the organizational setting, particularly when such ambiguity is reflected in the inability of the administration to formulate a new definition of the confidentiality principle.

The problem of determining ethical behavior on the part of the professional is complicated by the fact that most, if not all, ethical decisions are not a simple matter of choosing between right and wrong. The issues are not black and white when a question of professional discretion and ethics come into the picture; it is more a matter of choosing one good at the expense of another.

There has always been tension between opposites, between polarities, between disparate values resting on either end of the continuum of personal convictions and the collective ethic of society. For example, the perennial controversy still exists when the interests or rights of the individual contrast to the demands of society; the good of the individual versus the interests of the group or community, or even of another individual member of society; and the objective well-being of individuals as weighed against their right to manage their own lives and make their own choices.

When practical, real-life considerations are being made, the professional may at one time give greater emphasis to one or the other value in each of these dichotomies. Attempts to synthesize these values will not always be successful; nonetheless practitioners are responsible for making ethical choices and from this professional injunction, there is no escape.

REFERENCES

Campbell, C. Preventive measures by psychologists against malpractice suits, *California State Psychologist,* August 1977.

Congdon, C. Professional issues, *The Association for Advanced Training in the Behavioral Sciences*, February 1979.

Emerson, E. *Toward a General Theory of the First Amendment.* 72 Yal L.J.877, 918 (1964).

Klin, T., Gurstein, A., Hymon, E., & Navran, L. Ethical practices, *The Association for Advanced Training in the Behavioral Sciences, February 1979.*

Ostan, W. Unionization of the military: Some legal and practical considerations, *Military Law Review,* Summer 1977.

Robie, W. The teaching of professional responsibility to federal government attorneys: The uneasy perceptions, *Military Law Review,* Spring 1978.

Siemer, D., Hut, S., & Drake, G. Prohibition on military unionization: A constitutional appraisal, *Military Law Review,* Fall 1977.

Ethical Reflections On The Notion Of A Hippocratic Oath For Psychologists

CHAPTER 16

GIACCHINO V. SARNO

ETHICAL REFLECTIONS ON THE NOTION OF A HIPPOCRATIC OATH FOR PSYCHOLOGISTS

16

Giacchino V. Sarno

Inherent in the notion of an Oath for Psychologists is the presumption that psychologists are practitioners of a true healing art, and are themselves individuals who have the requisite intellectual and moral fitness. There are many physicians who would deny that psychologists meet either of these criteria. The following gives us some idea of the low regard in which psychiatrists generally hold psychologists:

> He [psychologist] is the mechanic without tools, the chauffeur without a car, the magician without his magic wand. His trademark is exactly similar to that of the orthodox psychiatrist, and being powerless to use any of the latter's additional medical modalities, zealously guards his tangential role in medicine. . . often using the title "Dr." as a prefix to his name and rarely the more explicit Ph.D. as a suffix, as though he is ashamed to admit the true identity of his title. . . . The psychologist is a hamstrung, pathetic individual who somewhere along the line missed the opportunity to study medicine and adopted a more pragmatic approach to his desired medical identity, with less obstacles (Schwitzgebel & Schwitzgebel, 1980, p. 233).

This is a generalization that does damage to the reputation of psychologists, and, ironically, serves, as do all such arrogant diatribes, to frustrate the efforts of those who would work toward better understanding between psychologists and physicians.

The fact that the diagnostic skills of psychiatrists are no better than those known to psychologists has not influenced state legislatures. For example, the majority of states do not grant psychologists the right to hospitalize patients. Neither do the lawmakers know that chemotherapeutic agents prescribed by psychiatrists routinely are not exempt from the pharmacological rule of thumb that all such agents not normally endogenous, induce side effects. In passing, we may note two: debilitating Parkinsonism secondary to phenothiazine management, and shortterm memory impairment secondary to electroconvulsive therapy.

Psychiatrists are embarrassed to admit that neurobiochemistry is a very recently born science, yet on the basis of it they claim superior knowledge. The actual reason that psychiatrists continue to argue that ECT is "appropriate" for certain cases is that they lack such refined knowledge of neural function that would allow development of a more effective and less risky procedure.

As a research biophysicist, I have often wondered why psychiatrists should be so concerned with a finite number of ECT subjects experiencing profoundly debilitating side effects. Electrochemical potentials with which the brain's neurons and glial cells operate are in the range of microvolts to millivolts; ECT potentials are on the order of tens of volts; i.e., on the order of 10,000 to 10,000,000 times higher than the brains own electrical parameters. Physicians are not necessarily exempt from the pleasures of vanity.

May I suggest that physicians assign psychologists the title "tolerated health professionals?" As a case in point, recently I attempted to have an individual admitted to a hospital—a 28 year old male, whom I found wandering on the beach, dazed, disoriented, talking of suicide, and of his divorce, in an alcoholic stupor, with deep open non-healing lacerations on both feet, contusions on his face, and no awareness of these injuries. The emergency room medic on duty gave this individual three Thorazine injections, and then, quite summarily, lectured him, "Alcoholism will kill you if you don't stop drinking. . . ."

I broke in and explained to the physician that the patient had no history of alcoholism (I had called his estranged wife, who so indicated), but began drinking seven weeks before, on the occasion of his divorce initiation; that though he was clearly in a state of alcoholic toxemia, this was due not to chronic alcoholism, but to drinking occasioned by psychological trauma.

I added that whenever you have a case of profound reactive depression, complicated by substance abuse, and accompanied by suicidal ideation, with no social support available, you have someone who should be hospitalized. The emergency room physician's reply was, "Look, psychiatric problems aren't accessible when somebody's drunk; they don't teach you psychologists the right things in school." I replied quite matter of factly that he was entitled to his diagnosis, but that I intended to maintain mine as well, not because of the psychological variables he wasn't considering, but because of medical variables of which, as a professional biologist, I was not unaware. A stab wound victim was rushed in at this moment and the doctor excused himself with the comment, "Excuse me but I have *sick* people to take care of."

We may as well admit that medicine maintains a certain ambivalent prejudice with respect to psychologists. On the one hand, where *sick* people are concerned, the psychologist is considered incompetent. On the other hand, where references are needed for scholarly medical publication, or teachers for psychiatry classes, psychologists are acceptable.

Lawyers are afflicted with a similarly obvious ambivalence. When it serves their purpose, they call psychologsts into court; when the psychologist's presence in court threatens to serve their opponents' interests, they are fond of discrediting, in a sporting manner, everything the psychologist says.

Perhaps, I would suggest, there is no reason to believe that psychologsts are inherently less morally fit than their medical and legal bretheren. Accordingly, we cannot maintain that psychologists lack the moral fitness that physicians would specify as a requirement for taking the Hippocratic Oath.

Indeed, we might wonder whether or not physicians' tendency to omit psychological dysfunction from the category "sickness," represents a lack of both intellectual and moral fitness on their part. This would apply mainly to physicians who are aware of psychosomatic interactions, but when pushed do not admit to being adherents of the new holistic approach.

There are no scientific grounds upon which anyone can validly assert that mental illness does not exist, or that purely psychological intervention is useless in alleviating psychic pain. Given this much, we can see that the art of a psychologist is indeed a "healing art," no less than the surgical techniques of physicians.

Since the psychologist's art is indeed a healing art, and since we cannot presume that they are morally unfit, both of the criteria identifiable as necessary for qualifying psychologists to take the Hippocratic Oath, are met. Hippocrates might suggest that we drop the terms which refer to drugs and operations, which is easy enough to do. For the word "drug" we can substitute "counsel," for the word "operation," "procedure." A copy of the Hippocratic Oath, so modified, appears at the end of this chapter.

I don't think Hippocrates would take issue with practitioners who heal the mind, by using their own minds. After all, Hippocrates was a Greek, who lived during the period of Milesian and Ionian philosophy. During his life (460-376 B.C.), Hippocrates witnessed and helped develop a philosophical movement in which Homeric mysticism gave way to a more harmonious balance between rational (which meant something like our "spiritual" to the Greeks) and empirical methods. Hippocrates would not categorically dismiss the possibility that mental factors and physical factors are indissolubly interconnected. In fact, one of the main ways that he differed from his predecessors was that he realized the importance of the environment and of the unity of interrelationships that characterize the human organism (Sirks 1964).

I suspect that physicians might offer only two other kinds of criticism with regard to psychologists taking the Hippocratic Oath. The first criticism psychologists should expect would be the accusation that psychology is not itself a sufficiently mature science, and because it is not, any pledge on the part of its practitioners to implement it, must be seen as premature and likely to cause more harm than good. The second kind of argument would be the childish demand that the Hippocratic Oath is *their* oath, and that psychologists should go and get their own. Neither of these criticisms, I am suggesting, can be rationally or morally supported.

The fallacy in criticizing that psychology is an immature science is that in order for this to be a criticism, Medicine compared against an absolute standard is itself perfectly mature. We must see, if we are indeed, any of us, scientists, that no science has ever yet achieved perfection. Science is authentic because we cannot dismiss its continuing perfectability, and cannot in good conscience deny mankind whatever measure of good our relative imperfection allows. We can see that if the criterion of appropriateness for taking the Hippocratic Oath were the absolute excellence of knowledge, Hippocrates could not have originally proposed it, and no modern physician could take it.

The Hippocratic Oath is not a scientific statement; it is a moral statement, which depends rationally only on the perfectability of man, and his knowledge, and upon those aesthetic and spiritual urges which give us this knowledge.

Science, as man currently practices it, has an epistemic status such that faith, morality and man's intuition are subjects that its language cannot encompass.

Someday, when the physical sciences and the social-psychological sciences have come to rigorous philosophical terms with one another, humankind may be able to ground its faith, and understand its love, with knowledge. That will be the day when science means something altogether new to culture, the day when every person will realize directly the operation of a single purposiveness in the whirling orbits of electrons and in the headlong flight of human consciousness through time and space. It will be the day when all psychologists may read in their history of science the first experiments and theories that confirmed A.N. Whitehead's epistemological principle of the "fallacy of mis-placed concreteness" (Whitehead, 1964). Physicists already know that the full significance of Whitehead's principle, which recognizes the manner in which compartmentalization of knowledge frustrates perception of its continuity, has yet to be realized. Physicists know already, because quantum theory and general relativity, and especially the recently developed marriage of these two theories, namely quantum geometro-dynamics, demonstrate the absolute interconnectedness of all of matter and energy, and the further dependence of all physical processes on the co-existence of perceiving (rigorously *participating*) beings (Wheeler, 1962).

The Nobel physicist Eugene Wigner (1967) says in his book *Symmetries and Reflections*, that at the center of the Universe we may find not a glittering mechanism, but magic. What kind of magic does psychology look forward to discovering?

It is significant that nowhere in the APA code of ethical standards do we find the words *love* or *wisdom*. With regard to Whitehead's caution against misplaced concreteness, and for that matter Godel's Theorem, which states that the possible extent of information exceeds the state of given systems content according to organization at a given time, how should we evaluate Behaviorism's claim that scientific psychology can be, as Skinner specifies, "value-free?" What can we make of Humanistic psychology's emphasis on *individual* responsibility when the presupposition of any ethical system is the absolute connection between the acts of all individuals? Why are there more physicists investigating ESP (psi phenomena) than psychologists? Because physicists have heeded more seriously Albert Einstein's admonition to use their imaginations at least as much as their reason, and have developed theories which do not categorically dismiss the idea of a process of absolute intercommunication between separate regions in Being?

Is it a coincidence that, simultaneous with the report that primates (chimps) can be taught to use language, Skinner had to report that "language" was not what the chimps had learned? What unsupportable prejudice is there hidden in psychology's adherence to Bridgman's "operationalism?" Why should certain orthodox doctrines of psychotherapeutic theory continue to maintain, in its static form, the principle that therapeutic success depends on an absolute impartiality and non-directiveness on the part of the therapist's conscious efforts? How much longer will psychology, which ought to be the science which, compared to other sciences, has less prejudice with respect to psychic reality, continue to see man as a "glittering mechanism?" When will psychological theory formally propose and affirm the magic of the human spirit itself? When will psychology, to which physical scientists look for answers about the psyche, start the task of recharacterizing its theories so as to bring them into line with consciousness itself? When will psychology become an ethical science?

Psychology, like every branch of scientific inquiry, must reserve Ethics, with a big E, for that criterion which we must yet seek to develop, that criterion which will enable us to form rational judgments about the ethical, with a little e. Ethics, with a little e, can be developed on the basis of current and prevailing social standards. Ethics, with a big E, for which we might want to substitute the term "wisdom," cannot be developed unless the "ethicizing" person (to borrow Waddington's term) asks questions that transcend the scope of what is actual, in order to uncover that which is potential in mankind (Waddington, 1960).

Though we need not concern ourselves with the anticipatable criticism from physicians that psychologists should get their *own* Oath, which they should somehow develop from their own ethics—as if Ethics has a different source for different practitioners of healing arts—it is nevertheless the psychologist's duty, as a scientist and as a person who claims any ethics whatsoever, to examine critically the extent to which given systems of ethics such as the APA Code, may be at cross purposes with Ethics. This means that psychologists have to recognize that their ethical propositions and the theories of human nature deduced from their scientific knowledge upon which these propositions are inevitably based, are subject to improvement.

To drive home this point, let us examine for a moment the APA's Code. Nowhere in the 10 Principles of the Code can I find explicit mention of the term Ethics. The term "prevailing social standards," however, appears frequently, and it should give us pause that along with dependence on this notion of prevailing conditions, there is no mention of a criterion against which we might judge which prevailing social standards are indeed Ethical, and which not.

Accordingly, a military psychologist can, without deviating from the APA Code, refuse to offer (violate?) the safety of privileged communication. Or would there be a deviation from Principle 3, which says that psychologists should be aware of the possible impact upon the quality of their services by their conformity to or deviation from prevailing social standards? We can see here that the Code lacks the kind of internal consistency that it might otherwise have.

Suppose that one has a military patient, up for promotion, with three children, who needs to talk about his abhorrence of killing, or of the guilt he suffers from having killed. Would the psychologist be acting truly Ethically if he were to tell this soldier's Commanding Officer? Should we consider as Ethical, procedures the psychologist might employ to alleviate the soldier's anxiety in order that he might forget about not wanting to go into combat? Herbert Marcuse (1966) has warned of the tendency of psychologists to become the unwitting lackeys of authoritarian interests unknown to the public at large, and of the fact that information provided to the public via the mass media gives equal time to both information and mis-information but no time to specifying a means for telling the two apart.

Does psychology so fear Wittgenstein's condemnation of abstract representation with regard to ethical propositions, that it fails to see the need for developing language which can express the realm of the Ethical? In agreement with C. H. Waddington, Michael Polanyi (1962), and the whole of continental Existential and Phenomenological philosophy, I must answer yes.

It is no coincidence, from the perspective I am advocating, that under Principle 4 of the APA Code, regarding Public Statements, we find no remarks concerning the possible desirability of an Oath. We hesitate to affirm publicly our ethical convictions because psychology itself holds fast to an epistemology that dismisses the subjectivity of ethical propositions in favor of a purportedly more reliable empirical objectivity. The moral consequence of holding that knowledge cannot be gained from human subjectivity, which is indeed holding to the most metaphysical of propositions, is that aesthetics and spirituality must vanish.

From my point of view, a view that cannot dissociate scientic from moral knowledge, the most fundamental problem with the APA Code is that it does not invite the psychologist, as the Hippocratic Oath does the physician, to consciously seek punishment for transgressing the very ethical propositions that it specifies. Nowhere in the APA Code do we find a statement even remotely analogous to the final sentence of the Hippocratic Oath:

> Now if I keep this Oath and break it not, may I enjoy honour, in my life and my art, among all men for all time; but if I transgress and forswear myself, may the opposite befall me.

I submit that the APA Code, because it contains no statement like this, lacks the most important Ethical principle of all, that of promising responsibility to one's fellows. And for this lack alone, not to mention the Code's lack of manageable length, I recommend that we substitute in its place the Hippocratic Oath.

Ethics, with a big E, because it requires that we seek the good without regard to prevailing conditions, necessarily asks of its adherents that which ethics, designed on prevailing conditions, need not ask: the courageous willingness to suffer the charges of subversion and the reality of danger to one's own life.

A question that psychologists must ask of themselves is whether or not they too suffer from a kind of "functional fixedness," a myopia, with respect to what should be the limits of the human spirit, and what principles of their science unnecessarily restrict the horizon of the possible, to the detriment of their art, and those who would benefit from it.

Christopher Lasch (1979), expressing the view of a growing number of social-psychologists, argues that advanced industrial society has prematurely socialized human beings, with the consequence that people's moral sensibilities have been left to atrophy and wither at the altar of conformity and productivity.

Perhaps if psychologists were willing to take an Oath, they would serve as an example for other people, whose latent moral and intellectual sensibilities would be stirred, re-awakened, and brought to flourish in the world. Let us turn to our science, and ask of it the ultimate questions. Since we are endowed with the freedom to choose, let us choose to take an Oath in which we proclaim the highest ideals that our searching science can reveal.

I would not suggest an Oath if I did not intend to take it myself. I recommend that any graduating or already practicing psychologist may, in confidence about the rightness of his or her act, take the Hippocratic Oath, before their family, friends, or, in the absence of an available or willing audience, before the wind, the sky, and one's self. (See Oath, as proposed, on following page.)

REFERENCES

Lasch, C. *Haven in a heartless world*, NY: Basic Books, 1979.

Marcuse, H. *One dimensional man,* Beacon Press, 1966.

Polyanyi, M. *Personal knowledge*, Chicago: University of Chicago Press, 1962.

Schwitzgebel, R. & Schwitzgebel, R. *Law and psychological practice,* NY: John Wiley & Sons, 1980.

Sirks, M. *The evolution of biology,* NY: Ronald Press, 1964.

Waddington, C. *The ethical animal*, Chicago: University of Chicago Press, 1960.

Wheeler, J. *Geometrodynamics*, NY: Academic Press, 1962.

Whitehead, A. *Science and the modern world,* NY: New American Library, 1964.

Wigner, E. *Symmetries and reflections*, Bloomington: Indiana University Press, 1967.

THE HIPPOCRATIC OATH FOR PSYCHOLOGISTS

I swear by whatsoever I hold most sacred that I will be loyal to the profession of Psychology and just and generous to its members; that I will lead my life and practice my art in uprightness and honor, that into whatsoever house I shall enter, it shall be for the good of the sick to the utmost of my power, holding myself far aloof from wrong, from corruption, from the tempting of others to vice; that I will give no counsel, perform no procedure for a criminal purpose, even if solicited, far less suggest it, that whatsoever I shall see or hear of the lives of any persons which is not fitting to be spoken, I will keep inviolably secret. Now if I keep this Oath and break it not, may I enjoy honor, in my life and art, among all persons for all time; but if I transgress and forswear myself, may the opposite befall me.

Giacchino V. Sarno

The Editors

THE EDITORS

EDNA J. HUNTER is the Director of the Family Research Center, United States International University, San Diego. Formerly she was Acting Director and Head of Family Studies at the Center for Prisoner of War Studies, Naval Health Research Center, San Diego. Dr. Hunter is a licensed Psychologist in private practice, a Fellow of the American Psychological Association, and the author/editor of seven books and over 80 journal articles/book chapters on a variety of topics, including sleep, dyslexia, prisoners of war, hostages, stress and coping, military families, and ethics and law. Recently at the American Psychological Convention in Anaheim, she was designated "1983 Distinguished Military Psychologist."

* * *

DANIEL B. HUNTER is an attorney at law, practicing in San Diego, California and Adjunct Professor, United States International University. He is a Certified Law Specialist in Family Law and a well-known authority on military law. He has lectured on various aspects of family and military law to both the legal and the lay communities, and serves, when needed, as a temporary judge of the Superior Court of the State of California, County of San Diego.

Cases Cited

Anclote Manor Foundation v. Wilkinson, Fla., 263 SO.2d 256 (1972).

Bellandi v. Park Sanitarium Ass'n, 214 Cal. 488, 6 P. 2d 508 (1931).

Bennett v. Jeffreys, 40 N.Y.2d 543, 356 N.E.2d 277 (1976).

Bernstein v. Board of Medical Examiners, 204 C.A.2d 378, 22 Cal.Rptr. 419 (1962).

Berry v. Moench, 8 U.2d 191, 331 P.2d 814 (1958).

Colorado State Board of Medical Examiners v. Weiler, 157 Col. 244, 402 P.2d 606 (1965).

Dugan v.

Ferrara v.

Grosslight v. Superior Court of Los Angeles County, 72 C.A.3d 502, 140 Cal.Rptr. 278 (1977).

Hammer v. Rosen, 7 N.Y.2d 376, 165 N.E.2d 756 (1960).

In Re Lifschutz, 2 C.3d 415, 467 P.2d 557 (1970).

J. B. v. A. B., W. Va., 242 S.E.2d 248 (1978).

Kent v. Whitaker, 58 Wash.2d 569, 364 P.2d 556 (1961).

Landau v. Werner, 105 Solicitor's Journal 1008 (1961).

Lassiter v. Dept. of Social Services, 452 U.S. 18 (1981).

McGowan v. McGowan, Pa.Super., 374 A.2d 1306 (1977).

Minnesota ex rel. Pearson v. Probate Court of Ramsey County, 309 U.S. 270 (1940).

Morra v. State Board of Examiners of Psychologists, 212 Kan. 103, 510 P.2d 614 (1973).

Mullen v. United States, 263 F.2d 275 (1958).

O'Connor v. Donaldson, 422 U.S. 563, 45 L.Ed.2d 396, 95 S.Ct. 2486 (1975).

People v. Peak, 66 C.A.2d 894, 153 P.2d 464 (1944).

Powell v. Risser, 375 Pa. 60, pp A.2d 454 (1953).

Index